RAISE THE BAR

HOW TO PUSH BEYOND YOUR LIMITS & BUILD A STRONGER FUTURE YOU

BEN ALLDIS

RADAR

First published in Great Britain in 2023 by Radar, an imprint of
Octopus Publishing Group Ltd
Carmelite House
50 Victoria Embankment
London EC4Y 0DZ
www.octopusbooks.co.uk

An Hachette UK Company
www.hachette.co.uk

Distributed in the US by
Hachette Book Group
1290 Avenue of the Americas
4th and 5th Floors
New York, NY 10104

Distributed in Canada by
Canadian Manda Group
664 Annette St.
Toronto, Ontario, Canada M6S 2C8

ISBN 978-1-80419-017-3

A CIP catalogue record for this book is available from the British Library.

Printed and bound in the United Kingdom

Typeset in 12/19pt Sabon LT Pro by Jouve (UK), Milton Keynes

10 9 8 7 6 5 4 3 2 1

Publisher: Briony Gowlett
Senior Editor: Pauline Bache
Designer: Rachael Shone
Assistant Production Manager: Emily Noto

With thanks to Matt Whyman

This FSC® label means that materials used
for the product have been responsibly sourced

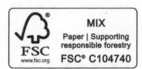

To anyone looking for a toolkit for living
a happier and healthier life.

Let this book be your call to action to take back control,
become your own coach, unleash your untapped
potential and continue to 'Raise the Bar' for yourself.

CONTENTS

INTRODUCTION: WHAT IS RAISING THE BAR?

We are capable of so much more than we believe.

All too often, we grow up to define ourselves by limitations. We tell ourselves we can only run so fast, jump so high, achieve a certain exam grade or settle for that comfortable rung on a career ladder. When we discover that some boundaries are there to be broken, it can be shocking, and yet deeply empowering. As humans, it helps us to feel alive.

As a Peloton instructor, my role is to endow people with the tools they need to rise to their full potential. It's easy to think that all that this is about is breaking into a sweat and getting into good shape (there's no doubt that physical fitness is a key pillar to living a healthy life), and yet I believe there's so much more to it than that. Our mental welfare is just as important, as is our social and spiritual health – and taking care of them begins with fostering a positive mindset.

By taking good care of ourselves on every level, as individuals and in our teams, we are equipping ourselves to raise the bar in our lives. From pursuing lifelong ambitions to facing unexpected challenges, it means we're giving ourselves every chance of coming through stronger and wiser for the experience.

I wrote this book as a wake-up call – for me as much as anyone I can help. We are all shaped by our experiences, and making sense of that can be a source of great strength. I wanted to understand the components that informed my outlook and the values they have taught me, and to show how this process is available to us all.

This book is not intended as a purely practical guide but rather as a means of thinking about our place in the world so we can learn from our experiences, build on successes and face forward with hope, courage and love. Ultimately, if we can look back knowing we put our heart and souls into everything we did then surely that is a life well lived? And if you're on board with that to begin, then let's ride . . .

PART 1

LET'S GO!

A bold vision is responsible for advances, breakthroughs and pioneering human achievements throughout history. It's how people change the world.

CHAPTER 1

ON THREE . . . TWO . . . ONE

*Our values are our bedrock, the platform that
we stand upon when preparing to raise the bar.*

I was a quick baby.

According to my parents, I shot into this world faster than my three sisters. I know birth isn't a race, but while growing up I was always oddly proud of that. It seemed to set the course for the rest of my life.

As well as being swift out of the blocks, I was long in limb and torso. My parents are quite tall and it seemed like I had inherited more than my fair share of those genes. Did this give me a notable advantage as a newborn? Well, I was standing unaided within my first year and then riding a bike before my peers were toddling. I guess I wanted to get cracking. I was too young to realise life is there for the taking, yet on some instinctive level, I seized every opportunity to be active.

By the time I started primary school, in my home town of Royal Tunbridge Wells in Kent, I towered over everyone else. I had no sense that it gave me a physical advantage. I just played with my friends like a normal kid and wondered why I would often be described as 'boisterous'. Once, at a school sports day, I lined up with my classmates to have a go at the unusual, quintessentially Kentish welly wanging contest (literally throwing a wellington boot as far as you physically can). Taking it in turns, each of us stood with our backs to the chalk line on the grass, then chucked a boot over our shoulders with all our might. Most contestants were lucky to actually launch it behind them. Several were rewarded with a clonk on the head. When it came to my attempt, I not only cleared the few metres that a boy from the year above had just achieved, but my welly sailed well over the playing field fence.

Despite my obvious welly-throwing capabilities, and realisation that my physique was a competitive advantage, I wasn't superhuman, just a boy full of enthusiasm who ricocheted through each day like a pinball. I imagine I must have been quite a handful; but my parents rose to the challenge, perhaps because my dad, in particular, understood.

Before settling into a career and starting a family, my dad had shown real promise across a range of different sports. He played district football and cricket and grew up playing golf in the same team as Paul Way and Jamie Spence, two guys who went on to become successful professionals on the European tour. Even when work and married life took over, his passion for sport of any kind stayed with him and made him come alive, and that was very evident to us as kids. Like so many fathers, Dad, I'm sure, hoped that his interest would rub off on his offspring. His first two children, my sisters, Jenny and Emma, enjoyed swimming, dancing and netball, but sport just didn't spark them with the same passion that they had for their other, more artistic interests fostered by our mother. My younger sister, Sophie, was the same and by the time we joined the Alldis junior squad, only one of us lit up completely at the prospect of playing football. So, based on our shared love for sport, from cricket and rugby to golf, but football above all else, my dad and I bonded, and I became his pet project.

'—*What was that, Ben? Pathetic! Come on!*—'

Touchline dads are a common feature of junior football. For some, seeing their children play brings out their inner José Mourinho. Mine just never stood back. From kick off to the final whistle, my dad would bellow at me like a Premier League manager whose multi-million pound signing had failed to deliver. If another kid messed up, Dad would let it go like he hadn't noticed, yet, even when the action was on the far side of the pitch from me, he'd still have something to say about my position. Now, my dad is a good guy, one of the finest, and he has always had my best interests at heart. Even so, as a five-year-old rushing after the ball with the rest of my teammates, I was mortified by his constant criticism of my abilities.

My dad never missed a match. Not only that, but he also became so invested in me as a player that he started helping out in running the team. Langton Green Community Sports Association is still going strong today, in fact, and he's a trustee now. In the past 25 years, or so, the club has grown to see thousands of kids like me come through the ranks and Dad's much admired and respected, known for being very kind to all the young players. It's just, back in those early years, he reserved all the tough love for me.

'What went *wrong*, Ben?' he once asked me on the drive home from an away game. 'I can't believe you missed that goal—'

'But Dad,' I said, exasperated, 'I scored three!'

The fact was I could have been player of the match and he'd still have found something about my performance to pick apart. I knew Dad meant well and yet it left me wondering just what I had to do to achieve the standard he expected. Maybe he thought I could take it, knew that I wouldn't crumble in the fact of criticism. The result: I concluded the only way to get Dad off my back was to become a better player.

To his credit, my father gave me every opportunity to improve. In his golden days, he had himself played in goal and was still a really decent keeper. So he decided to help me and, rather than make do with a couple of sweatshirts in the back garden, we built a goal out of timber.

'Let's see what you got,' he'd say as he took his position, inviting me to shoot. I faced him from the designated penalty spot, as he banged his gloved hands together.

Now, it's fair to say that when it came to scoring, most dads would probably be generous with their young sons or daughters. As a reward for effort alone, they might let a few goals in on purpose. My old man gave me no such break. Every time I struck the ball, he'd react like the outcome could decide the FA Cup Final at Wembley Stadium. With lightning-fast reaction times, he'd dive to one of the four corners to foil my attempt at a goal and then roll it back for me to try again.

There was no choice. If I was going to stick it in the back of the net then I would just have to improve. So, that's exactly what I did. After school, whatever the weather, I took myself outside and practised my penalty and free kicks, placing the ball on the spot and picking a corner of the goal as my target. Over time, my placement improved as much as the power of my shot, until eventually, when my dad faced me, I stood a decent chance of beating him. It meant when I did plant one in the back of the net, I celebrated like I really had just earned a trophy. While it might have been a dispiriting experience in the early days, eventually I found it deeply rewarding. Had Dad just let me score from the start, removing the challenge altogether, I wonder now if I would have got bored, eventually giving up.

But football wasn't our only shared sport, there was tennis too. If summer holidays are supposed to be an opportunity to switch off, my father had other ideas. Instead of flopping by the pool or beach with the rest of the family, he'd insist we find a court and play. I was always up for it, even though my opponent served with the same determination that he summoned in goal. When I was very young, he would beat me in straight sets. Over the years, however, I rose to the challenge. Eventually, I would win a point or two and even steal a game. It was a rare moment, and a sweet one that would see me punching the air. Even so, Dad didn't call it a day so we could unwind with my mum and sisters. 'Let's play another set,' he'd say, as if the last one hadn't counted, and I'd smile to myself because I knew how much that meant to us both.

Each year, even in the blistering heat of the day, our time on court grew longer and longer. The unspoken rule was crystal clear to me: we would finish when my dad finally won by a set. If I took another, we would just go again. I guess I could have let him beat me on purpose – if only so I could grab a drink and go for a swim. By then, however, the attitude to winning, obviously inherited from Dad, had become my guiding force.

When I expanded my sporting interests from football and tennis to the running track and found myself pushed to my limits by my coach, I have my dad to thank for the fact that I didn't resent it. I'd already been conditioned, if I was told I could do better, to not take it personally or walk away feeling like I couldn't cut it. All I wanted to do was prove to myself, and to those who believed in me, that I had what it took to be among the best. That didn't come from a place of arrogance: I never once expected to win without first putting in the work. I was just driven by determination, no matter how tough the challenge I faced. And that has stood me in good stead throughout my life.

From an early age, I recognised that sport would be central to my life. I was only following in my father's footsteps after all and I understood just what was behind his passion. Dad was born with a condition called lymphangioma, which caused cysts to form on one side of his face. He underwent a series of operations to remove the cysts and rebuild the affected area. It was considered a success, but I'm sure that, as a kid, the whole experience must have knocked his confidence massively and made him a target for bullies. Dad's own grandfather was an inspiration to him: he had lost a leg in a car accident when he was young, but that never held him back from living life to the fullest. And that was an early introduction for Dad to the concept of resilience. In the end, it was sport that saved him. With a flair for football, Dad discovered he was treated as an equal on the pitch by those who picked on him elsewhere, and his competitive spirit began to burn bright.

When his dream career as a professional sportsman failed to take shape, Dad didn't despair, however. Instead, at just 16 years old, he went to work in the back office of a bank. It was the lowest rung job, but as he saw it, there was only one way to go from there. Despite leaving his sporting ambitions behind, my dad found himself working alongside people in that business who loved to talk about rugby, golf, football and cricket as much as he did. It worked to his advantage when he bonded with an investment banker over a round of golf, leading to a job offer at the guy's firm.

Dad eventually reached the trading floor where he bought and sold currencies. With security on his side, he got married, settled down and started a family with my mother that resulted in my three sisters and me. I grew up in the 1990s when working as a city trader demanded a flash, brash character and the ability to negotiate deals with a phone pinned to each ear and, to me, Dad just didn't seem the type. While he donned a smart suit for work, at home his true self shone through – he was a bit of a scruff. Mum would cut his hair and he wore clothes for comfort without really caring about appearance. But he forced himself to dress up to be a trader, that ruthlessly competitive environment suiting him down to the ground. That fierce determination, commitment and sense of hard but fair play that he had learned on the football pitch stood him in good stead for a successful, more than 40-year career in the City.

Rugby was another sport that Dad adored. Many of his colleagues played for amateur teams like Wasps and Harlequins, in the days before the sport turned professional, and so the firm fielded a team that performed at a high level. As a squad member, he was in his element. With cricket, golf and tennis thrown into the mix, it's fair to say that my father pursued both work and play with passion, and as a family man he was keen to instil the values that served him so well in those fields in me.

No matter how I played, Dad was vocal about it from across the field. If I was going to calm the criticism coming from the touchline, that meant making the most of my physical size and the pace advantage this gave me. It wasn't about some natural-born skill – I really did tower over my teammates and opponents! I was pushing six foot in my later years at primary school – in squad photographs, I looked completely out of place. I learned to show up for matches with ID because I was often asked by the referee to prove my age. But on the pitch, my height advantage meant I could plough through players or outrun them because my legs were that bit longer. I played on the wing, sometimes up front and, slowly but surely, I found that commitment to keeping my dad quiet also led to goals and match wins.

Above all, I discovered I liked the buzz that came from playing to the best of my abilities. Throwing myself into a game from start to finish made me feel good. As well as bringing results, it also earned me attention from other teams. I joined squads with better players. By then my default response was to keep improving so that I became indispensable.

As well as my biggest critic, Dad was my unofficial coach, mentor and driver. We were a team of our own in some ways. As much as he drove me onwards, he also never let me forget my roots. Even when I had progressed to play at county level and was considering a career as a semi-professional player, Dad would badger me to come back and play for Langton Green's under-18s whenever I had time. I like to think my dad was proud of me and wanted to show the other players how far they could go, but, to be honest, he was probably just fixed on the win.

My three sisters enjoyed sport, too. It just wasn't with the same passion that bordered on a way of life which I had. Dad shuttled them to netball, no doubt hoping one of them would fall in love with the game and present him with another work in progress. Instead, their interest fizzled out. It was my mum who tapped into their creative side. An accomplished potter, and the perfect counterbalance to my dad's competitive side, she encouraged them to explore the arts. While their short-lived attempts to learn an instrument sounded more like scrapping cats to my young ears, my sisters found their feet and voices when it came to singing, dancing and theatre. Under Mum's guidance, they joined workshops and courses that brought out the best in them. The only downside was I had to join them. While Dad took me under his wing on a Saturday and Sunday, during weekdays it was Mum who called the shots.

'I can't leave you home alone,' she said when I first protested. 'I've signed you up as well.'

Standing on stage, squinting under the lights, was not a place where I felt at all comfortable, however. Unlike the pitch or the athletics track, I felt awkward and exposed. While it was good to spend time with my mum and sisters, delivering lines to an audience was not something that came naturally to me. But as Mum quite rightly refused to leave a small boy alone in the house, I just had to learn to make the most of it. At the time, performing in any shape or form felt like the last thing in the world I wanted to do. Now, I realise that I picked up skills that would become central to my way of life.

In a household with three sisters, I was quite comfortable in female company. Unlike those boys I knew who grew up alone or with brothers, I didn't feel the need to show off or be different around girls. I enjoyed their energy. My sisters liked to talk and were quite open about their thoughts and feelings. So, rather than be that boy who bottled up his emotions, I followed suit. Mum was always there for me in this respect. By all accounts, I was one of those inquisitive kids who had a question about everything, and she always found time to answer. I also knew that I could open up to her if something was troubling me. I've no doubt that my dad would have listened had I gone to him with a worry or a problem. Like so many men of his generation, however, I just wasn't sure he'd understand how to respond. 'You know what he can be like,' Mum would say with great affection. So, while my dad instilled in me a drive to win, my mum was there to remind me that it was OK to feel sad if I lost, or felt lost. It was just one more thing that brought home just how great a team my parents were when it came to giving us a solid start in life.

There was one other individual who played a formative role in guiding me into adulthood though – my father's father. Sometimes it felt like my grandfather was my greatest fan. I spent so much time with him as he lived locally. He was a pretty competitive guy, just like my dad and me, but he also listened. He loved to hear about everything I was doing.

We played a lot of board games together. Chess was a firm favourite, but because I was his grandson, rather than his son, he gave me plenty of scope to just enjoy the game rather than press for the win. Those longer games also meant we could talk in depth. As well as chatting about what I was getting up to in school and sport, he would keep cuttings from the local newspaper of my progress on the football field and running track. That meant so much to me and, over time, we formed a really close bond.

My grandfather liked to tell me about all the travelling he'd done over the years. That really sparked an interest in me, marking the start of a lifelong passion for expanding my horizons just as he had. When I joined my school's World Challenge expedition to Mongolia and China – a three-and-a-half-week adventure designed enable us to learn and grow as global citizens – he wanted to know every last detail of my experience, and I loved sharing it with him.

In being so close to my grandfather, I could see where my dad got his commitment to pulling a team together at Langton Green. My grandfather was a religious man, but through my eyes it was the social aspect of church that saw him attend on a regular basis. He was in his element when it came to being around people and helping them to get the best out of each other. He was an active man, who played tennis and golf right up until the day he died. Unlike Dad, it wasn't about winning or losing for him. He just wanted everyone to be involved in the same game and become stronger together, and I admired his commitment to something that so clearly completed him. Outside the church, he was the glue that showed our family how to pull together and stay close. My grandfather passed away when I was in my early twenties, some time before I would find my own community of like-minded people who would give me the same buzz that my grandad got from helping people to get the best out of themselves and each other. I miss him hugely but I hope I have made him proud.

*

WHAT MAKES US TICK?

'Who am I?' It's a question that we all ask ourselves at some point in our lives, and the answer is never the same for everyone. Each and every one of us is unique, after all, and that's rightly reflected in our responses. It means there is no textbook answer and that can be challenging. It's also an opportunity to settle upon a definition that could prove enlightening and a chance to get to the heart of who we are.

Why is it so important? Because understanding ourselves forms the foundation for our lives. It informs what we represent and how we relate to the world around us. It fuels both confidence and purpose in whatever we choose to do. We're talking about our core identity, and that runs deeper than our appearance or character. It's about the qualities in life that embody who we are, which we can call our *values*.

From honesty to integrity, a calm and positive approach to life or pure passion and commitment in everything we do, our values are a unique combination of personal qualities that get to the heart of what we represent. It's not a question of picking and choosing them to suit a certain situation. Even though it can take time for our values to take shape, if we can recognise their role in our lives, they become ingrained in the core of our being.

Our values are our bedrock, the platform that we stand upon when preparing to raise the bar. So, let's take this time to ask ourselves some fundamental questions.

WHAT IS THE *YOU* EXPERIENCE?

A performance coach once asked me a simple but searching question: 'What is the Ben Alldis Experience?

'How would someone describe you to one of their friends who doesn't know anything about you? What are the key parts of your identity and values that people would use to describe you to someone you didn't know?'

'A mix of everything really,' I finally replied, somewhat sheepishly. Eventually, after talking things through at length, I refined my definition to sum up what my coaching style represented. So, what is the Ben Alldis Experience? It's where my identity, core values and behaviours align. It's about finding happiness and personal reward through setting and achieving goals that are both realistic and enduring.

In a world in which we're encouraged to smash records and crush the competition, my focus is on finding space away from the crowd to understand myself, to connect with like-minded people and to live my life to the fullest by setting my own definition of what that looks and feels like. Whether you're faced with illness, a tough year at work or day-to-day frustrations, my coaching will help you build the physical and mental strength to move through challenges with confidence. In essence, I'm about building resilience and longevity into your life.

While this answer is specific to me as a Peloton instructor, I believe we can all benefit from asking ourselves that same question. It's not something we consciously put to ourselves on a regular basis, and it *should* be tough to answer. There *shouldn't* be a simple answer because we are complex creatures. In distilling ourselves to our core identity and values, however, we can then rebuild knowing what's underpinning it all. It takes time to figure out what we stand for, and not just to answer a question about our particular experience. We're not born with core values, like our organs, but over time they can become as essential to our lives as our heart and lungs. Like most people, I wasn't aware of my values taking shape as I grew up, but now I look back and can see those formative moments. From playing football with my dad on the touchline, which encouraged me to be determined, to recognising the importance of kindness in watching my grandfather connect with his community, I can count the individuals who shaped the values I hold today. But of course, like many of us, I wasn't always aware that I would carry such core values into my adult life. I just knew those people had made an impression on me. Whether it's family members or close friends, teachers, trainers or colleagues, even teams and social tribes, we can all identify figures in our lives whose core values we absorbed and then nurtured as our own.

Our core values can also evolve over time. Meeting new people, working for and with different organisations, experiencing other cultures and opening ourselves up to alternative ways of thinking can shape who we are and fundamentally inform our outlook on life. Most companies I have worked for have had a set of company values that they encourage their employees to uphold. Each of these businesses have shaped the way I approach my personal core values. Culture is the set of behaviours and practices that evolve from the values and mission of the company. It reflects the way the leaders and employees act even when no one is watching. When leaders and employees act in alignment with core values, it is a reliable indicator of a good culture.

Experience – the way we respond to certain situations – is another means by which we acquire or shape our values. I never liked seeing players missing out on being picked for a team, whether for a kick about with mates or a formal selection for a squad. At first I just felt sorry for them, but that instinct turned to compassion as I grew older – something I also came to respect as a quality in others. We learn by trial and error, of course, which often comes down to 'trialling' questionable values before recognising from experience that they don't work for us.

We all have different stories. No one else has lived the life you have lived. No one else has seen the things you have seen – or knows what it feels like to be you. No one else has experienced certain situations like you have. This makes it such a personal process when it comes to identifying the core values that guide and inspire us. While the outcome can only reflect the individual, let's consider the most effective methods to explore what makes us who we are.

IDENTIFYING OUR CORE VALUES

A core value is a principle that should inform and guide us through life. It can underpin everything from our character to the way we take on challenges. Our values aren't something that we pick off a shelf because they sound good. They exist within us, even if they remain unrecognised by us.

Imagine peering into a mirror that reflects the principles in life that are non-negotiable for you – a kind of human source code that shapes and informs your views, beliefs and actions. What are your core values, and are you using them to improve the quality of your life and your work? Here are six of my core values to give you an idea:

Positive Mental Attitude – Good energy will attract good energy.

Work Ethic – Step up, face challenges and take risks.

Love – Be a reliable, loving and trustworthy partner, friend, employee and son.

Gratitude – Turn what we have into enough. Being grateful for the people we love, the environment around us and the opportunities on offer to us.

Integrity – Be true to yourself and true to your word.

Leadership – Lead by example and empower others.

Now, let's start the process of identifying those values that are central to you. Below is a range of questions and a list of commonly held values. Answer the questions and pick five values that ring true to you – or nominate your own if that helps to reflect who you are.

What matters to you most?

What is a non-negotiable in your life?

What are the characteristics of a good person?

What is the driving force that is going to allow you to live your best life?

What are some characteristics you don't like about people?

What's a value that is opposite to these characteristics?

- ❏ Achievement
- ❏ Ambition
- ❏ Collaboration
- ❏ Creativity
- ❏ Dependability
- ❏ Empathy
- ❏ Enthusiasm
- ❏ Excellence
- ❏ Family
- ❏ Fun
- ❏ Integrity

- ❏ Happiness
- ❏ Leadership
- ❏ Growth
- ❏ Making a difference
- ❏ Optimism
- ❏ Popularity
- ❏ Stability
- ❏ Thankfulness
- ❏ Wellbeing
- ❏ Wisdom

Pause for thought

The chances are, you made your selection based on instinct. This is often an effective means of putting a name to long-held values. At the same time, it's easy to flatter or even undersell ourselves. That's why it's important to allow time for your chosen values to settle in your mind. It's a chance to be honest with yourself, and make changes where necessary. Consider it a period of refinement as much as reflection, and an opportunity to feel confident your values are true.

Consult and consider

We know that dialogue helps us to make sense of our feelings. You can apply the same to your values under review by turning to someone you trust – a close friend, colleague or family member – and inviting their insight and opinion. In order to maximise the return from such feedback, however, it's essential to bring self-awareness to the table. In my view, that is key to the self-development process.

It's vital that you can feel confident that whoever you approach will provide an honest assessment and be constructive in their criticism. You might want to share your selection from the list above – or a similar one – or first ask them to nominate five values that sum you up. Consulting those who you respect about your strengths and weaknesses can be hugely impactful to becoming your best self. The key is to keep an open mind about whatever they share. Allow yourself time to reflect, or work to refine those values that feel central to you. Ultimately, only you can decide what feels right, but it's another chance to sharpen and sculpt qualities that, once embraced, can serve to help you make the most of life.

What we're establishing here is our identity as seen through the filter of our guiding principles. Recognising our values is a vital first step on our growth journey. It feels good to know what qualities define us. It helps build our self-confidence and allows us to set our sights on new challenges with purpose and strength.

Ultimately, however, our values are meaningless unless they're reflected in our behaviour . . .

PUTTING OURSELVES TO THE TEST

One key purpose of having defined values is that they can hold us to account. If they accurately reflect who we are, then every moment of our existence should be consciously aligned to them.

For example, someone who believes that generosity lies at the heart of their being will express that naturally at every opportunity. It's a source of consistency in their life and also a source of pride. There's no pretence or concern about how they might appear, which removes a great deal of stress at a stroke. What's more, they can feel confident that such guiding principles will inform how other people will view them.

There is so much power in finding who we are in this world. The actions that we choose define who we are and how others see us. It's important to unplug from the social construct. Find and live out your own truth. Keep growing. Keep embracing the evolution of your own personal identity and core values.

Our identity and core values are something that we grow into through experience. For example, I spent much of my teenage years and early twenties painstakingly projecting a certain image of myself: the sporty type.

Even if I didn't buy into the 'alpha jock' mentality that was often prevalent before and after matches, this was my tribe. It gave me an identity at a time when I was still on the journey to working out that an active life could also be a compassionate and caring one. Eventually, the lessons learned from experience, along with a sense of maturity, helped me to establish the values that informed how I live my life. How do I know? Because my behaviour and the people who I decided to spend time around fell into lockstep with my guiding principles, and that's an evolution open to us all.

So, having developed a list of values for yourself, now is the time to challenge them to see if they stand up in real life. How? By actively monitoring your behaviour and being honest with yourself – being true to yourself. Just be sure to allow some time to let your behaviour play out. You can't make realistic judgements based on a short sample period – and there's no rush here to draw conclusions. Simply live your life and register honestly if your values lie at the heart of it all.

IDENTITY / VALUES / BEHAVIOUR

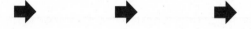

Ideally, our behaviour reflects our values, but if we're falling short we must ask what needs to change. Sometimes, our guiding principles can be genuine and yet we allow our standards to drop in the way we behave. We're only human, after all, and laziness, complacency and other self-destructive tendencies can creep in. Even so, we can also take responsibility for it; behaviour can be changed, after all. If you really believe that leadership is a value true to your heart, for example, yet you've been ducking opportunities, now is the time to level up.

At the same time, if your behaviour doesn't align with your values then perhaps it's because the values you've identified need reviewing. It's the ultimate stress test and can reveal a great deal about our strength of character. Nobody wants to face up to the fact that they're not as courageous as they'd like to believe, but owning that and working to identify what truly guides them is a commendable quality in its own right. It's also the surest way towards reaching that point in which our behaviour is a true reflection of our core principles. Then, everything we do in life aligns with our values and radiates from that point. In turn, that allows us to find peace with ourselves, build confidence, aims and ambitions, and seek purpose in life.

A review of this nature shouldn't be a one-off life event. In a business, quarterly reports allow companies to monitor, respond and optimise, and that's something we can also do on a personal level. It allows us to think smart and feel confident that the right strategy is behind us at all times.

WE CAN BE HEROES

In identifying our values, it can be useful to look to people we consider to be role models. They inspire us, after all, and if that encourages us to be better human beings that can only be a good thing. My grandfather is someone I admired very deeply. I am sure that his deep-seated values underpinned his behaviour. His entire life was guided by his religious conviction and, though it's not something I shared with him, I admired the commitment and devotion behind it. I've no doubt at all that he informed the values I hold today.

I have also found myself looking up to people in my industry and in sport who I respect and admire, and this has permeated my own personal development. Having goals is one thing, but seeing someone else at a place you want to get to can be a motivating force. In casting our net wide in search of those role models and heroes, however, let's be careful not to be seduced by how people sometimes appear in public.

For some, it's tempting to behave in a certain way for an audience, and effectively signal virtues that play well, because they reinforce a certain profile. Influencers have a role to play in our world today in terms of showcasing lifestyles or brands, but often it's an act, and financial motivation dressed up as real life. There's nothing wrong with liking or admiring anyone for the way that they present themselves to the world, but it does risk inviting unrealistic expectations among those who look up to them. We often see this across social media platforms which, let's not forget, are a showreel of people's best moments. Ultimately, we can't know what people in the public eye are really like in private, which is why the best role models are those who we trust embody our core values and/or people we know and love.

THE COMPASS THAT GUIDES YOU

Getting our values down to a simple list is no easy task (although the prompts on page 20 may help you do so). It can take weeks, months or even years. It's a different process for everyone, but once you're on the journey, that internal compass begins to activate. By this I mean utilising your values as guiding principles here. It's not about where we're heading – in love, life or our career – but how we conduct ourselves along the way. As an experience, it can be as rewarding as reaching any destination.

Our values also serve as touchstones, so that when we're faced with a challenge or difficult situation, we can refer to them in working out how to respond. If loyalty is one of our guiding principles then no incentive will tempt us to walk away from our teammates, friends, colleagues or associates at a time when they need us the most – even if we have to remind ourselves of that fact occasionally. Isn't that, after all, one of the simplest measures in life that confirms we're living the best version of ourselves? Meeting that standard isn't always easy, but it should come more naturally if our values are at one with how we interact with the world on our journey through life.

Good values don't just ground our decisions and underpin our actions. They can also help us form deep connections with people, teams or even organisations that share them with us. It's often said that the key to a lasting relationship isn't about whether you have compatible tastes in music, TV, fashion and style, arguably surface-level similarities. Rather, two seemingly different people can come together from opposite walks of life, their deep bond forming over shared principles in life, making it unbreakable.

Only you can feel confident in your values, but if they're true to your core nature they should shine through. Think of that friend or colleague whose character you can sum up in a few positive words. It's easy because their values define them. It's about simplicity.

Ultimately, these personal values can help to set our sights on goals and challenges, targets and adventures that may at first seem beyond our current abilities. What we're talking about here is ambition, which is the subject for exploration in our next chapter.

RAISE THE BAR: MILESTONES

- The first step of self-development is self-awareness. Understanding ourselves forms the foundation for our lives. It informs what we represent and how we relate to the world around us.
- What is the YOU experience? How would people describe your character and personality traits in a short sentence to their friends and family? If you are not happy with the first answer you give here, what actions can you take to help change that perception?
- In refining the YOU experience, identify your values. We're talking about the qualities that are consistent throughout your life, that you embody by your behaviour and that can be used as the compass that guides you.

CHAPTER 2

AIMS AND AMBITIONS

Inner ambition is about being at peace with ourselves,
knowing that we stayed true to our values.

It's only natural that our dreams become more grounded as we grow up. As children, we all want to be astronauts or superheroes, kings and queens, but then reality bites and we set our sights on more realistic futures. That doesn't rule out dreaming big, of course. Ambition is a healthy quality when it's underpinned by a willingness to put in the work to make it happen.

As a boy, I wanted to become a professional sportsperson. That was the dream, and I wanted to make it happen. Early on, it seemed like football offered me the best chance. Over time, however, I came to realise that there is no easy path, and very few players actually make it to that level. Still, when a rare opportunity arose to progress from county level, I seized it.

From when I turned 11, I spent my summers at Chelsea and Arsenal training camps. Among my footballing friends, everyone wanted to be spotted playing at a grassroots level by the famous under-18 wings of the Premiership clubs. I was so excited to be training alongside some of the best youth players in my age group. At the same time, I was aware that very few young players who are invited to these training camps actually make it all the way to a professional career. The odds are massively stacked against you from the start and yet, when I was invited to join, I couldn't let insecurity stop me from giving it my best shot.

I had been invited to this camp after playing in a junior tournament. A scout had come to watch me, although I was only ever aware of my dad on the touchline, my default being to play to the best of my abilities so that he wouldn't yell at me quite so much. On this occasion, that earned me an unexpected bonus. I was thrilled by the approach, but oddly it didn't feel like a dream come true. For years I had been climbing through squads, based on my ability, and had also been invited for trials in rugby and track. It meant I joined the football training programme without losing my head about it. Through my eyes, it was another step up and I knew that, if I was going to make a success of it and go on to the real prize of becoming a professional footballer, then I had to raise my game again.

In a short space of time there, I learned a valuable lesson. In any walk of life, there comes a point in rising through the ranks when you're no longer among the best in the field. And it's a humbling experience. At training camp, I was among players who left me feeling distinctly average. It didn't dampen my commitment, but it was a testing time. Even when I felt that I had improved, it seemed like nothing compared to some of the other players.

I was reliant on my parents to drive me around a lot to attend various training sessions and trials, across many sports, and it ended up taking up most of their weekends. They were completely on board with it, but I didn't take their kindness, time and energy for granted. It weighed on my mind alongside a growing sense on the pitch that perhaps my path to becoming a professional footballer might run out on me. That decision was taken out of my hands. While some players progressed for another season, after a year or so many, like me, were thanked for their time but informed that they would not be invited back.

I was gutted, of course, and I guess that's only natural. I'd chased a dream and it hadn't worked out. At that young age, with no experience of such rejection, it felt like my world had come to an end. It took a while for me to recognise that I was just one of hundreds of kids who showed some promise, but nothing close to what would be required for a shot at a professional career. It was a humbling realisation, but an important one. Once I was over the feeling that my world had stopped spinning, I also knew that I needed to make sure I didn't dwell on the disappointment. Fortunately, I was at a time in my life when I had lots going on to help put it behind me. For one thing, I was just getting to grips with a new school, and that proved to be as testing as my time on the sports field.

The Skinners' School is an all-boys grammar in Tunbridge Wells. It was local to me, with a reputation for excellence. Above all, I wanted to go to the school because it was known for being really sporty. The main sports coaches at the time were an ex-Wasps player, a retired New Zealand cricket player and the former vice-captain of Somerset Cricket Club, and their teams usually crushed the opposition on the cricket field, the rugby pitch and everywhere in between. I saw it as a chance to pursue all manner of competitive sports at a high level.

The only catch, I learned, was that, in order to gain a place at the school, I had to pass the 11+ exam. An entry qualification based on academic performance, it meant I spent the best part of my final year at primary school gearing up to sit the examination. My school head questioned whether I would pass, which came as much as a shock to my parents as it did to me. I had always kept up with my schoolwork, yet now it seemed like that wouldn't be enough. To keep my options open and, possibly, to lessen the pressure of me not getting in, my mum and dad took me to open days at other schools. While I could see the attraction of some, compared to Skinners', they all placed less emphasis on sport. But, as if my dad was on the classroom touchline to keep me on my toes, I was determined to aim high even if it meant a lot of work to reach the level required.

We all face decisions like this early in life. Often they're steered by those who have our best interests at heart. My parents laid the foundations, but ultimately the decision on my future fell to me, and I took it seriously. Even though I was so young, I knew where I wanted to be. When the 11+ results came in and I learned that I had passed, it just reinforced my belief that I could go places as long as I put in the effort. I'd been determined to prove myself, and so, when Skinners' offered me a place, it felt like a step forward.

It was only when I started my first term at grammar school, feeling grown up and excited about the sporting opportunities, that I realised what a challenge I faced. I had worked hard to pass the entrance exam. For the sole aim of turning those papers and putting in my best effort,

I basically *trained* and *drilled* myself to punch above my academic weight. Then lessons began in earnest and I found myself outclassed by everyone around me. I went from being one of the brighter kids in my peer group to the kid who struggled to keep up. What's more, in that grammar school system, I found the emphasis on getting good results left me in danger of feeling like a failure.

Finding myself at the bottom of the class did not sit well with me. I felt like I was missing something that my peers all seemed to possess when it came to comprehension. They just seemed more on the ball than me. If I were being honest, I knew that at primary school I'd been so caught up with playing sport at every opportunity that I hadn't read that much. All of a sudden, this put me at a huge disadvantage. It knocked my self-confidence for sure, but I didn't cave. While it didn't feel good to be struggling when it came to tests, grading and end-of-term reports, I believed I could turn it around. For one thing, my classmates didn't seem to be naturally brighter than me. Many of them had been privately educated or received extra tuition in the holidays; they struck me as being 'book smart'. So, I just had to keep reminding myself that I'd always been able to deliver just as long as I did the work.

As a motivating factor, that sense of being at the back of the pack was enough for me to seriously get my head down in a bid to get to the front. I focused during lessons and made sure I understood the subjects we were covering in class rather than let it all go over my head. As a plan of action, it stopped me from panicking. Thankfully, I had sport to keep a sense of balance in my life. It meant I made the most of my time both in and out of school. As a result, term by term, my results began to improve. By extension, that helped me to feel like I was getting a return for the extra effort I had invested. I had earned it the hard way, having worked so hard in the school library and at home out of hours, which came down to wanting to prove myself. I could trace it back to the touchline, of course, where I first had to make a choice between walking off the pitch, in the face of criticism from my dad, or rising to the challenge. Now that the latter had become my default mode, it meant I could focus on what lay ahead for me rather than dwell on the past and wish I had tried harder.

Call it grit, the will to persevere or pure stubbornness – and I had my dad, and the generation preceding him, to thank for instilling this in me. It kept me focused and motivated. I also saw what happened to those who hadn't been challenged in the same way. More often than not, when faced with an obstacle, they crumbled. Some just seemed to give up when it came to schoolwork, while later a few found themselves drawn to making poor decisions in other areas of life. In school assemblies, we often heard about the importance of resilience and it seemed to me that it was a quality I had already developed. It felt like a superpower in some ways, and it didn't let me down.

In terms of my immediate goals, I wanted to do well at school. Beyond that, now that my chances of becoming a professional footballer had been given a reality check, I began to see myself following in my dad's footsteps. He was passionate about his work, and that rubbed off on me. The trading floor sounded so exciting, and that stayed with me as I came to make informed decisions about my choices of subjects at GCSE and A Level. I wasn't following a grand masterplan from the start, but slowly a big picture started to emerge. As it became clear to me that I was shaping up for a career in the City, that helped me proceed with confidence.

There came a point on the journey when I paused to review where I was heading. It was sparked by an internship. My dad arranged for me to shadow him for a month during the school holidays and I jumped at the chance. I only ever saw him head off to work ready to take on the day, and then return looking like he finally had a chance to power down. This was an opportunity for me to see him in action, to experience, first-hand, how it felt to be in the role that had become my career ambition.

It was not how I imagined it would be.

Dad had always painted a picture of the trading floor as an energetic and often dramatic place to work. Through the eyes of a schoolboy, however, it was relentlessly noisy, chaotic and often overwhelming. I liked the energy, but when it came to considering my place in it, I struggled. My dad literally came alive as a trader, whereas it left me with a feeling of menace; as if I was in a zoo where the cages had been left unlocked. In truth, I was overwhelmed by such a visceral environment, and that forced me to question whether it was really the job for me.

For a while, I told myself that I just needed to get used to life as a trader. Every day I shadowed my dad, however, I found the voice of doubt in my head growing louder. As my internship progressed, I had to wrestle with a looming conviction that I had gone down the wrong path. In my mind, I worried that I had made poor decisions about the choice of subjects I was studying. I was chasing qualifications suited to this field, such as maths and economics, and now I found myself questioning my end goal.

Fortunately, I talked to my dad about it. He acknowledged that the trading floor wasn't the same place it had been when he first started. It had shifted a gear and he had strapped in for the ride. It meant that, when a trade went wrong, he had to keep his nerve, maintain a front that everything would be fine and then metaphorically spill blood, sweat and tears to make that a reality. It came down to character and also explained to me why he was so adept at keeping his emotions in check. There was no room for anything but relentless confidence. I just wasn't wired in the same way. I was a thoughtful kind of person. I tended to weigh up things before acting, and there seemed to be a lot less time for that here. To my surprise, in chewing it through with my father, I realised that all was not lost.

I had expected him to tell me to man up. If I felt like I couldn't play to my best abilities here, I thought he would say, then I needed to try harder. Instead, having picked up on the fact that I was struggling to match the reality of his workplace with how I had imagined it, my dad encouraged me to take a broader view.

The trading floor might not have been for me, but I still had the ability to shape my future. If anything, he helped me to realise that my internship was a chance for me to review my plans and make changes before committing to anything. Despite my experiences in the City, I remained fired up by the world of finance. It also felt reassuring to know that Dad still believed in me. I just needed to find another way into the industry that suited my personality. I wasn't frightened of having to work hard: it was simply a question of finding the right position on the pitch.

Viewed in this way, the month shadowing my dad in what had seemed like the wrong fit for me, became a positive learning experience. It led me to move on from trading as a potential career path and focus on aspects of finance that required considered thought. As a result, my interests turned towards investment management and consulting. It seemed like a much better match to my character. Above all, it involved building trusted relationships with clients, and I really loved working with people. The more I looked into this field my confidence grew that I had finally found the right path for me. It meant I was able to look back on that internship with nothing but gratitude to my dad. He had shown me what I didn't want to do, and then supported me as I reviewed my options and refined my focus on just where I felt that I could shine.

*

AIMS AND AMBITIONS UNBOXED

When people learn that I'm a personal trainer, they often assume that means I'm out to smash my training goals at all costs. To be honest, if my sole ambition was to push myself to an extreme – as well as those who train with me – then before long we'd all end up burned out. That kind of full-on, uncompromising strategy works for some, but in my view it's not sustainable. It might lead to short-term goals, but I prefer to plan for the long term, as I strongly believe that's where we feel most fulfilled.

When I think about ambition, and what it means to me, I consider it in one of two ways. First, there is our outer ambition. We're talking about our drive for success, recognition, fame, power or wealth, whether it's for personal gain or public good. From childhood dreams to career goals, our outward ambitions can be big or small in scale. We might devote our entire lives to making a far-off ambition happen, or set ourselves a target of getting into shape within six months, or save to go travelling and see the world. From short- to long-term objectives, we tend to view our outer ambitions as a way of defining our place in the world.

Then we have what I call our inner ambition. We're talking about seeking to live our lives true to the values we've identified as our core ones. If I believe that kindness lies at the heart of who I am, for example, then my value ambition is to express that kindness in everything I do. The same applies to any value that we identify as central to who we are, from loyalty to commitment to fairness and equality, to courage and curiosity. It's an aspiration in many ways, and one that can hold us to account in the way that we relate to the people and the world around us.

Our inner ambition should enable us to reach a point where we can look back on our lives and then say that we lived it to the best of our abilities. It's also this ambition that can bring us lasting happiness and fulfilment. It goes beyond power, wealth, recognition or achievements. Inner ambition is about being at peace with ourselves, knowing that we stayed true to our values.

GROWING THE GOAL

We are all different in the way that outer ambitions take shape in our minds. When we're young, however, it's fair to say that most of us harbour big dreams. I wanted to be a professional footballer, in the same way that others saw themselves as superheroes or jet pilots. Unlike most kids, it wasn't just a fun fantasy that helped me to think about the future. I really did take steps towards that career. When that faltered, I turned my attention to other goals, but the experience still taught me to aim high, and I stand by that today.

In dreaming big with our ambitions, we set ourselves on a quest that can only test our limits and even encourage us to push beyond them. That doesn't just allow us to grow. A bold vision is responsible for advances, breakthroughs and pioneering human achievements throughout history. It's how people change the world. Even if we set ourselves ambitious objectives only to rethink along the way (because sometimes life steers us in a different direction), that initial ambition has still helped us to develop as individuals. We can still look back and take pride in the fact that we tried and feel stronger for the experience.

Outer ambitions can drive us from one challenge to the next. Our goals can be personal and professional in nature, and serve as stepping stones as we negotiate life. From turning a side hustle into a small business to becoming financially secure or able to provide for ourselves and others, our outer ambitions set up purpose and reward. They can contract and expand in scale as we see fit, and even take us in surprising directions.

At the same time, if we're clear about the values that lie at the heart of who we are, then our inner ambitions should be a constant guide in our lives. Here, our aim is to embody those core beliefs and use them as foundations for personal growth. If we start out aiming to be loyal, that becomes an inner ambition and we can apply it to everything we do. As a friend, partner, colleague, teammate or citizen, if we can earn a reputation for loyalty, then we have achieved something deeply meaningful. Not only is it rewarding for us, but it's a force for positivity, and we can put no price on that.

We need ambition to succeed. There is no point having a huge skill set if we don't have the motivation to go out and use it. That goal can be an incentive. It can remind us why we've making sacrifices and commitments, and that doesn't just apply to elite athletes, but anyone who has set their sights on achieving something beyond easy reach. In sport, very few people are prepared to put their lives on hold in pursuit of that medal or trophy, but when it's the focus for their existence, it becomes a powerful force.

My outward ambition as a coach is to help people transform their lives. I want to help others feel great by embracing health and fitness, which sets them up to make a positive impact in other areas of their lives. It's an aim that has evolved over time, until I reached a point in my life where it has become a heartfelt commitment.

A primary reason for this, as we'll explore next, is because my outer and inner ambitions have at last come together to support each other.

WHEN AMBITIONS ALIGN

Empowerment lies at the heart of my core values. I want to help and inspire others to fulfil their potential. It took some time, experience and maturity for this to become clear in my mind, even though it's existed in me from a formative age. As a team player in youth leagues, I'd always wanted my side to be firing on all cylinders. Over time, that extended to a general awareness in me that, with focus, support and passion, we all have the ability to exceed our expectations.

When my footballing goals faded and finance took shape on my horizon, it's fair to say that I didn't give much thought to my inner ambition. I wanted to follow in my father's footsteps and build a future in the City. My outer ambition took over, which was all about finding a career ladder that I could climb. I wanted the financial security, structure and certainty that a post in the finance industry could bring. As a student and in my early twenties, it was only natural to think about defining myself in terms of achievement, and even status. As I became more self-reflective, that changed. This is how our inner ambitions come into play. For some, that means finding themselves on a course in life in which their outer ambitions don't support their true values. I met plenty of City workers in this position. Their jobs demanded that they made money at every opportunity, and that could mean investing in industries such as oil or tobacco. For some, this clearly didn't sit well with their personal values. There was no way the work that fulfilled their outer ambition could also support their inner ambition.

It's perfectly possible to follow two different paths in terms of our outer and inner ambitions. I've no doubt my work colleagues would go home and find joy, happiness and fulfilment among family and with friends or by pursuing pastimes that served as an escape from their professional roles. We just have to ask ourselves if that's really the most fulfilling way to live our lives.

Of course, there are plenty of people in the kind of work who lean towards their outer ambitions (even if it's just a question of earning a living) and who devote their spare time to fulfilling their inner ambitions. We might be drawn to charitable causes or environmental and political campaigns to express our true nature or find meaning and personal reward in specific areas, from parenting to touchline coaching, a passion for travelling or a hobby that we adore.

For many, that clear division between inner and outer ambitions works just fine. Given the choice, however, it's always worth asking ourselves if it would be more rewarding to seek a path that supports both at the same time. If anything, that uniformity can only help to build a strong reputation. We only have to look at influencers who work with brands they believe in to recognise the power at play here. Working with stakeholders that align with their values creates credibility and promotes trust, whereas those who take on any endorsement purely for the financial incentive risk looking hollow and do little to sustain longevity in their field. Ultimately, if you're a kind person in both your professional and personal life, that has to create a positive impression to the wider world. It shows authenticity, which is priceless when it comes to everything from contentment to career development and prosperity.

Today, when I look back at the path I followed to arrive as a fitness coach and trainer, I can confidently say that my ambitions have aligned at last. I work in a role that rewards me on a professional and a personal level. I am motivated from the heart, and that brings an energy and positivity to everything I do. There is an old saying: find a job you enjoy and you'll never have to work a day in your life. Through my eyes, that showcases how it feels when our inner and outer ambitions come together. For me, uniting them across all aspects of my life is where true happiness lies.

DREAM BIG, THINK SMART

Let's consider our ambitions as a destination. We know that our outer ambition is about following a path that leads us to the place of our dreams, even if it's the highest office in the land or a first-place spot on a podium, and that journey is made all the more rewarding if it also embodies out inner ambitions. This raises a fundamental question, however. If our outer ambition is out of this world, exactly how do we get there?

First, it helps if our inner ambitions – our core values – align with that goal. Even if that destination changes as we go through life, which is increasingly common as communication and technology exposes us to ambitions or goals we might not have considered at a previous time, we can still ensure we're on track. If we're genuinely passionate because it chimes with our personal beliefs, that's effectively rocket fuel. It means we're committed to the ride and prepared to face all manner of challenges along the way. When things get tough, we never lose sight of that goal because it means so much to us on every level.

We're not just talking about career goals here. One of my central ambitions has always been to be a family man, alongside a loving partner who meets me at the levels of life that I want to live. This has become a driving force for me alongside my career pursuits. Ever since I was young, in fact, I have dreamed about inspiring my future kids, just like my dad and my grandad inspired me. In some ways it's a personal ambition, but the values behind it also drive every other aspect of my life.

Even if our inner and outer ambitions are aligned, it's worth noting that, if any goal we have is a long distance away, it's at risk of seeming unachievable. Setting our sights on space is a case in point, and yet every individual who makes it beyond the Earth's atmosphere started out with the same bold dream. So, how did they get that far? In every case, when it comes to big ambitions, we have to break that journey into manageable goals.

We don't need to look to the stars to see this strategy in practice. Ultramarathon runners often rely on an approach called *process over outcome*. Rather than thinking about running one hundred miles, which can seem overwhelming, they focus on not just one mile at a time, but often one footstep after another. In this space, runners tune into delivering their best at every moment in time. By reeling in their focus in this way, and effectively practising a kind of mindfulness on the move, the finish line no longer serves as a tortuous reminder of how much further they have to go to achieve their ambition. It becomes the reward for their perseverance and smart thinking.

A little thought goes a long way when it comes to pursuing our ambitions. As kids, we dream big without any consideration of how to get there. Then, when it becomes apparent just how much work, skill, resilience, dedication and time it involves, as well as all the barriers that stand in our way, we often turn our attention to goals that are easier to attain. This is a shame, in so many ways, as there is much to be said for harnessing that childlike optimism and then applying grown-up, considered thinking to the task. At a stroke, it can make the impossible seem possible.

So, let's look at the key points to consider when it comes to stress-testing any ambition. If we can establish a realistic strategy, no matter how out of this world it might at first seem, we can undertake the journey by following not just our hearts but also our minds.

TESTING THOSE AMBITIONS

Establish the goal

There is a difference between identifying our destination and working out how to get there. Begin by keeping it simple and put a name to your ultimate aim. For now, don't worry about how to make it happen. Bring out that inner child and dream big.

Do your ambitions align?

The great thing about ambitious thinking is that it tends to be driven by our values. When Apple's co-founders set out to create their first computer, it was effectively a product of their innovative spirit and passion for combining design with technology. Establishing an outer ambition that allows you to express core beliefs can only strengthen the commitment required to make it happen. Your inner and outer ambitions don't have to align, but if they do, it can only prove to be a more rewarding experience.

Work out what's involved

Take a practical approach to the project. From acquiring new skills to picking up experience, making new contacts and finding a way to work towards your goal, there could be a great deal to consider. Begin by brainstorming what's involved, then take time to order and refine that list.

Get energised

I thrive around people who are going places. As a coach, I find it inspiring to be in a room full of people with different ambitions in life. They could be running business start-ups or creative agencies, raising young children or seeking to improve their fitness. I love talking to them about their lives, challenges and objectives, and admire their resilience so much. It also opens my eyes to what's possible. No two people have the same goal and yet I find everyone's focus, enthusiasm and energy to be infectious. What's more, when we assemble for an early morning class, I feel as if we're feeding off a collective energy that helps each of us to become stronger when we depart to seize the day.

Assemble a support team

Behind every elite athlete is a crew of trainers, friends and family. They each play a vital role in helping that athlete fulfil their ambition, and the same applies to any walk of life. Now is the time to think about the people you need on your team, even if that just begins with letting loved ones know your plans. Chances are, you'll meet individuals along the way who can support you in fulfilling your ambition. It's here we should also consider the importance of a mentor, which is someone with the wisdom and experience to help guide, support and advise us when we need it. Just be smart about who can help, and grateful for their time and energy.

Consider a timescale and make it manageable

Much depends on the nature of your ambition, but it often helps to use time as a frame of reference. It can be a motivating force and a means of measuring progress: there's nothing like having a deadline. Perhaps you give yourself a check-in at one week, one month, three months, six months and one year. Then think about what is a five-minute action you can do today to get closer to your goal? Action creates progress. A five-minute commitment is a great way to overcome triggers, set small goals and achieve lasting success. By taking the first five-minute step to focus on yourself and your health, you can make great strides towards a healthier and happier lifestyle.

More often than not, five minutes turns into thirty minutes and so on.

Review your progress

Any journey you undertake in pursuit of an ambition will be transformative. You may pick up experience and new skills along the way, face unexpected setbacks and even opportunities that only open up *en route*. In this view, the smart move is to establish moments of reflection. It's about asking if your initial ambition is still just as important to you, or has the process of getting this far led you in a new direction?

Personally, I like to work with one-, five- and ten-year plans. It allows me to set up both short- and longer-term goals, with an opportunity at each point to take stock and consider where I'm heading in light of what I've learned along the way. In establishing your own ambition plan, just aim to build in those moments to look back on where you've come from before assessing the way ahead.

Embrace the quest

Whatever destination you have in mind, there are plenty of pathways to get there. In many ways, that's the beauty of pursuing a long-held ambition. Only you can choose the right course, and you have the ability to change and adapt it according to circumstance. Consider your ultimate goal as a beacon. When set up with care and consideration as much as passion, it'll always shine brightly to guide you, no matter what route you choose.

BEYOND AMBITION

As a final note, to close this Part, I'd like to encourage us to stop thinking about ambition in terms of failure and success. Not everyone with a childhood dream of becoming a professional sportsperson is going to see that become a reality. As I discovered, the odds are stacked against them from the start. We know that shouldn't stop anyone from pursuing such a goal if it comes from the heart. By breaking up the quest into manageable goals, it can become a rewarding process in its own right. At the same time, my early dreams to play sport at the highest level meant I was exposed to all manner of different experiences and exciting opportunities that ultimately steered my career path. Becoming a Peloton instructor wasn't a dream that I could have had as a kid, but I've arrived here as a result of those early ambitions in sport, and I've discovered it's exactly where I want to be. A dream is just that until we take steps to turn it into a reality. What's more, the act of setting off on that quest can only open up the chance to fulfil different ambitions that aren't just achievable but possibly also more rewarding.

RAISE THE BAR: MILESTONES

- It's important to recognise the difference between our outer ambition (a drive for success in a career or challenge, for example) and inner ambition (living a life true to our values, such as one guided by happiness, courage or equality).
- When our inner and outer ambitions align, they become a powerful force.
- Big dreams can become an enduring reality, if we think smart from the very first step and learn from the journey.
- Dream big, be smart and enjoy the quest along the way. There is no such thing as failure if you give something a go. The only failure is if you don't try.
- You may be doing a job in two, five or ten years' time that doesn't exist right now. Stay hungry to learn, stay current with technological advances and be open-minded with how industries and the world are developing.

PART 2

RHYTHM

By constantly striving
to build knowledge through experience,
the more we grow as individuals
and the more informed
our choices will be.

CHAPTER 3

MINDSET AND MOTIVATION

Life can throw challenges our way, but it's only by raising
our game to meet them that we grow and become more resilient.

There are times when a casual conversation can resonate deeply. Soon after it became clear to me that I wasn't going to become the professional footballer of my dreams, I had a chat with my dad, one which would go on to shape my approach to life.

At the time, I was devastated by the news that my childhood dream of playing football professionally was slipping away from me as I was not chosen to return to training for the next season, no matter how hard I had pushed myself. I had worked so hard to reach the highest standard I could, yet somehow that had not been good enough. So, I couldn't help feeling as if it had been one big sacrifice of time and energy for nothing. I had been the one to watch throughout my primary school years and, at such a young age, it felt like that attention would last forever. With commitment, I'd also known that I had natural sports ability: I could play at a high level in rugby or cricket, and my times as a runner meant I could be taken seriously as a track athlete. So when my golden ticket to become a professional footballer seemed like it had expired, it forced me to question if any kind of sporting ambition was worth the effort.

'You can't give 100 per cent to everything,' my dad told me in a bid to lift my spirits. 'You *can* fully commit and focus on one sport, and we'll totally support you in that. But if playing sport for fun is all you want, then you can still learn a lot along the way.' It was a rare moment for me to hear him talk in this way. At a dark time, it was just what I needed. 'As long as it makes you happy, that's what really counts.'

In my summers at training camps, I'd really struggled to find the time to play anything but football. I loved all sports, however, and so I made it work even though it left me exhausted. At one point, I was so run down that I picked up a bout of glandular fever. It really floored me, and our GP warned me that I should be careful in future. So, with my dad's advice in mind, I looked back, realising that in trying to play everything to the best of my ability, I had been compromising myself across the field. It seemed to take ages for me to recover from being ill, which was another sign that I needed to rethink my relationship with sport. The way to excel, as Dad had spelled it out, was by committing myself wholeheartedly to a single discipline. I only had to listen to the story of any successful professional sportsperson to recognise that rising to the top demanded the kind of commitment that prioritised one thing over everything else. I had that passion for football. But I could say the same thing about all the sports I played. Above all else, I really enjoyed just being active, I realised, and that's what settled it for me.

Rather than devote myself to one pursuit and place that above my schoolwork, friends and family, I decided I would simply embrace sport of all kinds because it made me feel good. That didn't mean losing my competitive spirit, but rather finding a way in which I could play for fun. Sport made me happy, so surely it would have a knock-on effect on all other aspects of my life?

Free from the pressure I had placed on myself to become a professional footballer, I threw myself into cricket and athletics at school. I even took up golf with my dad – which was striking for being the one time he didn't make it his mission to win but to chat and just have a nice time. And I played football on a semi-professional basis with Tonbridge Angels FC. This gave me a chance to enjoy it at a decent level, but without the stress of feeling like my future depended on it, and I thrived.

Dad also persuaded me to keep on playing for the team he managed, Langton Green, on a casual basis. He would often whisk me away after a Sunday morning fixture with the Angels so I could start a game with my mates in the afternoon, and I loved it. I put my heart and soul into every minute on the pitch, but did so with a smile on my face. That set me up for the school week, at a time when I was beginning to work my way up from the lower sets.

Even with the career pressure removed from the mix, I still liked to play hard when the opportunity arose. Rugby was a case in point, and I threw myself into being selected for the school team. Our coach had ruthlessly high expectations. He didn't take any shit and expected us to be top of our game every time we played and trained. We competed at a national level, against future professional rugby union players like Elliot Daly and Joel Hodgson. I was playing at the top of my game, and certainly building resilience thanks to the toughness of our coach but without the anxiety of having my career goals pinned to it. As a result, I loved every moment.

My dad's advice of playing for fun and being happy had such a positive effect on me. Having initially instilled that competitive edge in me, which I loved, he had also helped me to recognise that enjoyment can also be a motivating factor when it came to any pursuit. Until our chat, I used to become quite tense ahead of any match or track meeting. I was only young, after all, and was investing so much of my energy into sport that I felt like I couldn't afford to lose. At the time, I didn't know how to process pressure in a productive way. I was frightened of failure, and that led to nerves and excitement turning to stress and worry.

From the moment I started playing for enjoyment, that anxiety I'd experienced just melted away. I still retained the drive to win. I wanted to play to the best of my abilities. I just didn't have to go through that feeling of dread beforehand, and that helped me to feel so much happier. I never went through the same worries in school. When I reflected on this, I realised it was because I was chasing from the back of the pack rather than leading from the front. It meant I placed less expectation on myself. I just thought I'd give it my best shot, and then steadily began to climb through the ranks. In sport, being head and shoulders above my peers from such an early age, I felt like I had everything to lose. That fear of failure shaped my mindset until I stepped back from sport as a 'make-or-break' activity, just playing purely for the passion.

In that same period of time, during those early years at grammar school, the physical advantage I'd enjoyed over my peers began to close. As we hit adolescence, I found that everyone, from my friends to my teammates – and the opposition – were beginning to creep up on me in terms of height and build. I might have been an early developer, but that counted for nothing by the time I turned 16. Had I been stuck on the dream of becoming a professional footballer, I imagine this might have been devastating. Instead, as my focus had shifted to proving myself academically, it almost came as a relief.

With the playing field levelled physically in all the sports I enjoyed, it took away any remaining sense of pressure I felt to be the best at all costs. At the same time, I didn't just stand aside for players who had enjoyed a growth spurt. Of course, I still wanted to play to my best efforts, but if I couldn't outpace my opponents, or simply push through them, it meant I had to rely on skill instead of brute strength. And so, playing for fun motivated me to sharpen up other aspects of my game rather than freezing under the pressure to perform.

I see my school years in terms of two journeys. First, in sport, I stepped back from the top rank in order to have fun; second, in the classroom, I learned to apply myself in pursuit of better results. As time ticked by, and I left my dreams of becoming a pro footballer behind, it became quite clear to me that I was applying my energies to the right path. Having shadowed my dad at work, I had refined my career ambitions and that really helped to drive me. The trading floor wasn't for me, but I had become as interested in business as much as finance and wanted to work at the point where the two sectors came together. I knew that I couldn't just walk into a job. In a highly competitive field, I would have to shine as I did on the football pitch. That meant working my way through my exams and then a degree in order to gain qualifications that would help me to stand out. It was a long-term goal that demanded commitment: I knew where I wanted to be and what I faced to get there.

With an endgame in sight, I worked hard through school to sixth form. Like many kids, I found casual work to bring in some money. First, I had a job in a big retail chain, my first real experience of a public-facing job. Mostly I worked on the checkouts, learning the good, the bad and the ugly of customer service. I also worked my way up from a pot-washer to managing a front-of-house team at catering events, such as big weddings or parties. While I did it for the cash, it helped me realise what I enjoyed most: interacting with people, delivering a service and ensuring they had a great experience. It gave me an early taste of the kind of work in which I truly came alive.

Sport still played an important role in my development through this time and helped me negotiate teenage life without making too many poor choices or big mistakes. I was on good terms with most people in my year and would go to many of their gatherings and late-night parties with my team-mates. I think these social events were important learning experiences as a teenager and they were one of the ways that my friends and I bonded. However, there was no way my teammates and I were missing games or turning up to them hungover. It turned out that sport was the guiding force keeping my friends and me out of trouble. Drinking a lot or taking drugs just didn't really fit in with that lifestyle and, because I was considered athletic, that was accepted without judgement or mockery, although I was mocked for other things in the classroom.

Sport was so important to me that it even played a role in my dating life. As a pupil at an all-boys school, it wasn't easy meeting girls. Once or twice a year, the school would co-host a disco with the girls' school across the road. Some of the boys from my year didn't know how to relate to the opposite sex, either showing off or just acting like complete fools. Coming from a household with three sisters, I was used to female company and just found it a relief to be among them and I tended to hang out with sporty girls. Through my school years, I went out with a couple. It was fun, but nothing serious. In some ways, it felt more like we were teammates than boyfriend and girlfriend, and that was fine at the time. We had common ground, sharing priorities, juggling schoolwork with training. In short, we understood each other. We wanted to work hard at school, play hard outside it, but ultimately be happy within ourselves.

Of course, like any teenager, I didn't have it all worked out at the beginning. My competitiveness was a central driving force in my life, no doubt helping me to work my way up from the bottom of the class when my opportunity to become a professional footballer disappeared. Even so, there was only one place where I liked to be the focus of attention, and that was on the pitch. In school, I could be quite self-conscious when it came to speaking up or answering questions.

Since starting at Skinners', I had always felt that I processed information differently from everyone else. Initially I'd assumed I was just bad at reading and writing, but then I was diagnosed with dyslexia. In some ways, this helped me to feel more positive about approaching the challenge. At the same time, however, it made me a soft target for teasing and mockery. And growing up noticeably taller than my peers didn't help. At a time of life when I lacked confidence, it was tough being the one who literally stood head and shoulders over everyone else. This was reinforced one term, some time before everyone caught up with me, when the deputy headmaster faced a particularly talkative gathering one school assembly. He had asked for silence several times, only to be ignored, so set out to make an example of someone. I had been just one of over 800 boys chatting, but pretty much saw what was coming as his gaze swept over the rows in front of me and then settled on the tallest poppy in the hall . . .

'Alldis! *Get out*!'

As a hush fell around me, I had no choice but to stand up in front of everyone and make my way to the exit doors. My cheeks were hot with humiliation and also indignation – I had been one of the few pupils sitting quietly. It felt like punishment for being tall and did nothing to encourage me to draw further attention to myself.

In contrast, on the football pitch, the bigger the crowd, the better. I liked nothing better than sinking a ball into the back of the net and then celebrating with my teammates. In school, however, if all eyes turned towards me, I wanted to hide away inside myself. I felt so uncomfortable with the spotlight on me in the classroom. It was only when I reached the sixth form, however, that I realised this attitude was holding me back. In the first year of sixth form, we could apply to become school prefects. At that time, with university applications on the horizon, I was always looking out for ways that I could gain an edge. Getting involved in school life at this level seemed like something that would set me apart, but I knew that any boy in such a role would be expected to do some public speaking.

Up until then, I had only one experience of this for reference– I'd had to address my year group as part of a presentation. I'd been so nervous beforehand, and that peaked when I stood up to speak. I felt hot, sweaty and dizzy, and stumbled through whatever I had to say. My dyslexia didn't help, of course. It felt like my brain was moving at one speed and my mouth at another, and it went so badly that people mimicked me for days afterwards. On the pitch and the athletics track, however, I didn't have to do any talking and felt at home, yet I knew public speaking was something I had to master if I wanted to make the same impact on my world outside of sport. So, when I applied to become a prefect, I made a deal with myself. If I was successful, I would become comfortable with a social skill that basically terrified me.

The interview for the position of prefect was a serious and intimidating affair. I faced the headmaster and several staff members, and they basically grilled me about what I could bring to the role. I gave it my best shot, but left feeling like it had been a disaster. I felt like I had busked my way through so many of the questions, and only really came alive when asked what had motivated me to put my name forward.

'I believe in fairness,' I replied, meaning every word. 'If something isn't right then you need to stand up and do the decent thing.'

I really did hold true to my response. It's just the interview panel looked at me like I'd invited them to step outside for a fight. Still, when I looked back at the experience, even believing I'd probably blown my chance of becoming a prefect, I knew I had given it my best shot, so I had no regrets. If anything, it had been a learning experience, and it was the last time I faced an interview panel without feeling properly prepared.

Much to my astonishment, I was made one of four heads of house, responsible for representing a quarter of the school and motivating them to sign up to house events. It was such an honour. I wanted to make a difference and ensure that every pupil felt included and appreciated. When I told my grandfather the news, I felt like I was taking over the torch he had carried in terms of values for life. At the same time, I knew I would have to honour my promise to myself – to tackle the one component of the job that truly frightened me.

Even today, when I teach indoor cycling or deliver a talk as a motivational speaker, I carry the memory of how scared I used to be when it came to public speaking, when I first stepped out as head of house and my heart raced and my mouth went dry. What saw me through it was a refusal to be defeated. My first few attempts were pretty forgettable, but, slowly, speaking to audiences became a familiar experience. I learned to prepare what I had to say, with notes in hand if I needed them. Gradually, I discovered that I preferred to read the room with a loose structure in my mind and then just go with the flow. It was a skill, I realised, not a natural born gift, and required practice in order to improve. That was what drove me to stick with it, and I'm so glad that I did. Public speaking might once have seemed like the last thing I wanted to do, but it's served me well throughout my career and now I genuinely love it. Even so, I never want to lose sight of the sense that I'm stepping out of my comfort zone. It's a healthy part of the process, I believe, and helps to keep me on my toes, to strive to be better. Without it, I might be at risk of sleepwalking through a speech or workout at a moment when engagement is vital.

I was confident that the experience I picked up at school in public speaking would help me when it came to applying for a place at university. True to my sporting roots, I aimed high from the start and applied for a place at Oxford University. I built myself up for the application interview, ready with everything I intended to convey, predicting how I might feel in that situation and with strategies up my sleeve to make sure I came across in the best way possible. But I never made it to an interview as my initial application was met by a straight rejection from Oxford. I realised it was time to get realistic. I had done well at school, relative to when I started out at the bottom of each set. Even so, I hadn't climbed so high that I could take my pick of the top-flight universities. I received offers, but they were conditional on grades. So, when my A Level results landed slightly below what had been predicted, I worried that my end goal of a career in the City might have slipped beyond reach and I was keenly aware of how competitive it was. Employees could select from candidates with shining CVs, and feeling sorry for myself wasn't exactly a selling point I could add to mine. If I wanted to keep my dream alive, it meant I had to impress when face to face with any panel that I came across in my future.

Even though I didn't get the opportunity to interview (or its accompanying red-faced moments) I knew that the build-up and preparation that I had put into my proposed Oxford interview would serve me well for the future.

I was relieved when an offer from Leeds University to study Economics came, however, I couldn't help but feel a pang of disappointment. My school had consistently pushed us to be the best. It was an uncompromising attitude in some ways, which made it hard for me to see most of my friends head off to their first-choice universities. Leeds looked good, based on my visit to the city when I went for the interview. It just wasn't considered to be a classic route into the City. It was like working hard to make it to the final of a football tournament, only to lose just before the final whistle.

Which is when I wobbled.

It was that classic case of not feeling good enough, even though I'd given it my best shot, and it knocked my confidence. I tried to put on a brave face. I was about to leave home and start a new chapter in my life, but, in truth, I was gutted. A small voice inside me questioned if it was worth spending three years studying at a university that hadn't been on my radar until my results arrived.

While Leeds wasn't my first choice, and tested my motivation to keep on pushing, it was the best thing that could have happened to me. My degree course was challenging and, with plenty of sport to keep me focused, I fell in love with city and university life. Having come from a quiet town in Kent, Leeds felt like a whole new world. It was exciting, with so much going on culturally. I found myself surrounded by people from all walks of life, and it broadened my horizons no end.

By the end of my first term, it felt like all the hard work I had put into going to university was paying off. Even if the outcome surprised me, I wouldn't have had it any other way.

*

MINDSET MADE EASY

We hear a great deal about 'mindset' today. It's a term we often throw around without truly understanding what it means. This is a great shame, because, with clear understanding, our mindset can transform our lives.

In a nutshell, we're talking about the way we feel when we naturally respond to a challenge. All sorts of factors can come into play, of course, from what's involved in undertaking it to our reason for taking it on in the first place and the reward on the other side. We could be talking about anything from applying to become a prefect at school, climbing a mountain or asking someone out on a date. Ultimately, when we're tested in some shape or form, it reveals our true nature. It can make or break this testing time. It's also something we can control and use to our advantage. That's what we call our mindset.

There are two ways of looking at what is basically our attitude towards obstacles or opportunities. A fixed mindset is one in which a person seeks reasons not to embrace a challenge. This could be due to a lack of motivation or self-belief and can be established through habit or certain patterns of behaviour, and seriously work against us through life. We're talking about taking the path of least resistance here. It's the easy road, but also one that doesn't give us the opportunity to shine. We just plod from A to B, and that's fine. It's just in doing so we sacrifice the chance to live up to our full potential.

With a growth mindset, however, we're prepared to take the

difficult path. It might require new skills, time to prepare or even involve a support team, but, with this viewpoint, nothing will hold us back – especially not ourselves. A growth mindset encourages us to seek opportunity rather than play it safe. Even if we don't succeed in our objective the first time, it allows us to learn from the experience – and to grow stronger from it.

All too often, we find ourselves defaulting to a closed or 'fixed' mindset, defining ourselves by our limitations instead of our potential. In terms of our attitude, we tend to think 'why me?', rather than 'try me!' It's also tempting to stay within our comfort zones, but over time they can become prisons without us even realising. We can change our outlook though and adopt a growth mindset. It doesn't require a course or a qualification. It's just about wanting to make positive change and taking small steps onto the path that builds confidence and takes us not just to the mountain tops, but beyond. Let's examine how to make that happen.

CLIMBING THAT MOUNTAIN – ADOPTING A GROWTH MINDSET

Be honest
Optimising our mindset starts with a period of self-reflection. We need to be crystal clear with ourselves about how we view challenges. We might possess a growth mindset when it comes to pursuing work opportunities, for example, but then close

ourselves off to our full potential in our personal lives. Everyone will have a different perception of their mindset. In establishing what that is – with absolute honesty – we can build a platform for change.

Be inspired

We look up to certain people for good reason. My focus isn't on individuals who wear the trappings of success, but those we truly admire because their behaviour and attitude shine out. They don't have to be famous. Ordinary people do remarkable things every day. Like my grandfather. If we open our eyes to their quiet achievements, we can recognise they possess the kind of mindset we all aspire to. At the very least, they can provide a template for us to establish a way of approaching challenges and obstacles in life that works for us.

Be bold

Very often, we talk ourselves out of taking on a challenge because there is a risk of failure or rejection. Nobody wants to learn they've been overlooked for the job they applied for, or get knocked back when they ask someone out. It's human nature, but then ruling ourselves out without even trying can only lead to one outcome – wondering what might have been.

It takes courage to embrace the risk of failure and rejection, and the key is to see it as a learning opportunity. We grow from our mistakes if we teach ourselves not to repeat them. It means we can go again with wisdom or a different strategy on our side, or simply use that experience to our advantage elsewhere. Yes, it takes practice to deal with missing out, but looking for the lessons takes the sting out of the tail. So, whenever faced with a challenge and our instinct is to pass, let's take a moment to remind ourselves that being bold is where it all begins.

Be smart

Possessing a growth mindset doesn't mean we should say yes to everything. It's about assessing any kind of challenge and working out what's required to stand a strong chance of success. Often, this means learning new skills or taking time to establish a strategy. It might also mean calling upon the help and assistance of others. In applying for a job, for example, it's always worth asking someone who works for the company what it's like in reality. That level of insight can inform not just whether you feel it's the right opportunity, but also provide an edge when it comes to the application process. Talking to a trusted friend or colleague on any level can allow us to find clarity in how we approach challenges in life – and ways that we can improve. All of these are options to be considered. This way, we can make informed decisions and take on challenges knowing that we're prepared.

It's amazing what a transformation we can make to our mindset using just these four tools of being honest, inspired, bold and smart. By being up front with ourselves about our attitude to a challenge, finding the courage to recognise that failure or rejection is a learning opportunity and then preparing ourselves to give it our best shot, we can confidently say that anything is possible. By removing the barriers that traditionally stand in our way and adopting a growth mindset, we can all go far in life.

EXPERIENCE IS EVERYTHING

As I've already shared, as a boy, I found it hard to deal with the slow realisation that I wasn't going to make the cut as a professional footballer. I had imagined myself playing in the Premiere League, so when that dream came to an end, I was incredibly disappointed.

It was my dad who picked me up, and he did so by giving me options. He encouraged me to think that I could still enjoy the game at a less competitive level. At the same time, with the pressure off, I could make time for the other sports I loved, as well as focusing on getting a decent education under my belt. In helping me to recognise that this path was right for me, Dad encouraged me to look back at my journey as a youth player and appreciate just how amazing it had been. OK, so I wasn't able to climb through the ranks to play at the highest level and I would never lift a trophy at Stamford Bridge or Wembley Stadium, but these things were ultimate goals. What really mattered, I came to realise, was the experience I'd enjoyed along the way. That's what had shaped my character thus far, and none of that would have happened had I stayed in my room and played video games – or given up when things didn't go my way.

This was a turning point for me in terms of how I viewed challenges. I stopped looking at the prize with regard to the outcome and learned to value the process instead. When it comes to focusing our mindset, it's an effective way to approach new objectives. It means there's always value to be had in the undertaking, even if we don't succeed at first in our main aim. This is how we grow as individuals, because every experience shapes us, allowing us to grow wiser and stronger, if we choose.

Let's say we train to run a marathon. If we all set off hoping to win or smash our personal bests, or PBs, what's going to happen if we start to drop our pace? With our sole goal slipping away, it would be so demoralising that our heart wouldn't be in the race any more. But what if we entered for the sheer experience? Sure, we could still push ourselves in terms of performance, but this way we might get to appreciate more – everything from the cheering crowds to the celebratory atmosphere. Regardless of our finishing time, we'd also have learned so much about ourselves. The medal might be a nice, shiny memento, but the value? The story of our entire race, including all the training that went into it. That bigger-picture view can only set us up, not just for future races, but also any aspect of our life moving forwards which demands resilience, focus and determination.

A practical way to broaden our experience is by embracing new opportunities. It can mean being open to conversations with different people, even if they don't share our own views or morals, and learning from diverse backgrounds and cultures. By constantly striving to build knowledge through experience, the more we grow as individuals, and the more informed our choices will be.

I believe a growth mindset is available to us all. The smart way to deploy it is by making the experience the reward in any challenge we take on.

MINDSET IN MOTION

But what happens if we construct a growth mindset with good intentions, only to find that we falter when faced with obstacles in our path?

As a fitness instructor, I am always meeting new people. My job is to energise and inspire, and that takes a confident, outgoing personality. I love the role, but still think of myself as an introvert at heart, the person who struggled with confident public speaking. Over the years, I've taught myself to overcome that instinct to hold back, simply because it's not in line with my aims and objectives in life. I want to connect with people and bring them together under a shared objective, and that never happens unless I step forward and introduce myself.

It's not uncommon to feel reserved or doubtful about our abilities when we're presented with a challenge. Sometimes this is down to our need to fully assess a situation before we commit, which is a positive quality. Very few of us would jump off a 10-metre diving board without hesitation. The human instinct for self-preservation, survival, would kick in, yet sometimes this can hold us back. I'm talking about situations in which we can minimise risk by making informed, considered decisions. That's the approach we need to embrace in order to summon the courage and focus required to make such a leap. It's the most effective way to stop us from hiding behind that natural response to something seemingly tough or difficult.

Once we've assessed what needs to be done both safely and constructively, and we're motivated in the knowledge that we can only grow from the experience, it's vital that we find the courage to step forward. That is the moment a growth mindset turns from theory to practice. In leaving our comfort zone behind, it's also when we meet our true selves.

As well as constantly pushing us to take on new challenges, a growth mindset can enable us to expand our knowledge. A hunger for learning is key here. Often, on finishing formal education we pull back or simply learn what we need for a particular job or task. This is a shame because the fact is our brains gain so much from a continued quest for knowledge, but we need to build this into our lives. Personally, I consider learning to be so important that it's become a vital part of my self-assessment. If I am expanding my knowledge base, I am growing. In the same way, as humans we exist with limitless potential. We are inherently curious. We like to play and push just to see how far we can go. It can become a means of defining ourselves, and this applies to anyone who has set out to break anything from a personal best to a world record. Ultimately, we can take ourselves in any direction, but in every case a growth mindset is the key driver.

There is another common moment in the real world that can put our growth mindset to the test. It occurs in all manner of situations, but effectively takes shape when a challenge we've embraced becomes progressively harder. We could be talking about facing setbacks or simply a moment when that path has become far steeper and more technical than anything we've encountered so far. It's one thing to take on a new challenge, but quite another to stay strong when things become tough.

I loved my early years playing football. Much of this was down to the fact that I had a physical advantage over my teammates. As I've detailed, I was taller and broader than most kids my age, even at primary school, and I used this on the pitch to become the player who caused most problems for the opposition. Inevitably at that age, it proved to be a honeymoon period. I might have been an early developer, but eventually everyone caught up with me.

As a result, my playing advantage began to retreat and it felt like I was going backwards. I was no longer head and shoulders over everyone else on the pitch. While I had worked hard to become a decent player, it suddenly seemed as if that had a sell-by date. Critically, I chose not to brood about it or resign myself to what felt like a demotion in ability and that's thanks to my dad's encouragement. Instead, I vowed to get better.

It helped that I had three sisters. We got along just fine, but, apart from the arts courses our mother signed us up for, I didn't really spend time with them. So, with nothing else to do – and with my dad concentrating his sporting hopes on me – I took my football into the back garden and practised. I took free kicks until I could pretty much score with my eyes closed and, when my dad was around, he'd join me to provide a presence in goal and challenge me for possession of the ball. I spent more time outside the house than inside. As a result, I raised my game. I became a better, more precise, player, and returned to being a threat to the opposition despite being no taller or broader than anyone else on the pitch.

It was a formative moment for me, not just as a footballer but also in terms of my mindset and motivation. It certainly set me up to knuckle down when I moved from primary to grammar school – and sunk from the top of the class to the bottom. The lesson: life can throw challenges our way, but it's only by raising our game to meet them that we grow and become more resilient.

A SHOWCASE FOR OURSELVES

We know that a growth mindset plus motivation can take us places. It's the means by which we ignite the touchpaper rather than letting it grow damp. We're talking about that 'can do' attitude. When combined with smart thinking about the skills and help required, it can become a formidable force.

In helping us to shine, of course, that positive attitude means that people will pay attention for all the right reasons. To illustrate this, just think about how we view people with a growth mindset. We're impressed by their energy and willingness to try new things, and, when that person has taken steps to research a challenge or acquire the skills required, it pretty much ticks all our boxes. Even if they fall short of reaching their goals, it's their enthusiasm and drive that earns our respect and even applause.

If we adopt that outlook ourselves, just think about what a positive impression that will make on others. A growth mindset fuels everything we do with a positive energy, and that can come to define us. When it comes to making an impression on people, it's a quality that they can only admire. In fact, it's more likely to attract people who share a similar mindset and are going places as well. A positive mental attitude can bring so much more than a sense of wellbeing. It has the ability to propel your whole life as those around you will be moving in a positive direction too.

When I look back on my early attempts at public speaking, my performance was shaky at best. Nevertheless, it was the effort I made that counted more than the polish. It also led to further opportunities for me to practise and refine my delivery, and that wouldn't have happened had I not volunteered and challenged myself to step up in the first place. In short, a positive outlook on life doesn't just lead to personal development. It encourages others to recognise you're someone determined to be the best version of themselves.

STRONGER TOGETHER

A growth mindset doesn't just benefit the individual. Collectively, it can be a driver for wider, positive change. We only have to look at successful football teams, businesses or civil rights movements to recognise the power that forms when people pull together to take on a challenge.

Before teaching class, I am met with people from all walks of life. Everyone is different. Some are fizzing with energy. Others are frazzled from parenting or a project at work, but looking forward to time out. Then we start the session, and I can sense every single person present commit to making the most of it. Some might be training for a triathlon. Others are simply looking to get into shape, not just physically but mentally. Their end goals may be wildly different; even so, everyone is united in their motivation and the mindset required to take on the challenge of an intense session and enjoy the buzz that comes from it.

I have no doubt that our environment can have a huge impact on our mindset. While everyone has to find their own mindset and motivation from within, a group environment can help to unleash it. If one person arrives for a session feeling down or distracted, it's very hard for them not to be lifted and swept along by the collective energy in the room. It's contagious! In effect, we're facing a challenge together and sharing the load.

There are also broader benefits that come from being strong together. Even if people are pursuing different personal goals, that shared mindset provides a foundation for us to forge new friendships. I have met so many interesting and inspirational individuals in fitness classes, as both a student and a teacher. Some have led to professional opportunities. Others have resulted in lifelong friendships. I especially love the fact that, at the end of a challenging session, everyone leaves with that positive energy we've created together, sharing it far and wide – the gift that keeps on giving.

RAISE THE BAR: MILESTONES

- Understand how you naturally respond to a challenge and make changes, if necessary, to transform from a fixed to a growth mindset.
- We can learn from experiences. Even if we don't succeed at the first attempt, the wisdom and skills acquired in the process can help us grow, go again or take on new ventures.
- Life is like riding a bicycle: to keep your balance, you must keep moving. Commit yourself to a lifetime of continued learning. The most valuable asset we all have is our mind and what we decide to put in it is down to us. Every day is an opportunity to learn something new and build a stronger future you.
- Find a group of people that challenge and inspire you, spend a lot of time with them and your whole world will change. Tackling challenges with other like-minded individuals can create a force that is greater than the sum of its parts. Alone we are strong, together we can be stronger.

CHAPTER 4

BUILDING ON EXPERIENCE

*Playing sport for pure enjoyment became an
effective means of taking care of my mental health
in a way that was fun and fulfilling.*

My degree gave me valuable insight into all aspects of world economics, from finance models and mathematics to politics, sociology, entrepreneurship, law, psychology and history. Without doubt, those four years of study equipped me with a broad range of knowledge for the industry I'd set my sights on even before university. If I look back at Leeds, however, it was the experiences of life outside the lecture theatre and library that gave me the practical and interpersonal skills that changed my life. Clubbing being a case in point.

For a kid from leafy Kent, the nightlife in Leeds blew me away. From freshers' week onwards, I regularly went out with friends to enjoy a few drinks, dance and meet new people. After dark, there was always something going on across a wide range of tastes and genres. For me, it was incredible to see the impact music and nightlife had on people. It brought everyone together in a space that freed them up to be themselves, and that was a revelation. For a kid still passionate about sport, I found this resonated in just the same way. From gatherings in low-key pub basements to the big venues in the city centre, I loved the atmosphere and the sense of release from the pressures of life. I also wanted to get involved behind the scenes. So, when the opportunity arose in my second year for me and a couple of friends to get involved in running an established club night, we seized it, without knowing the first thing about how to do this. As first-year students, we had been regulars at the event. It was popular, loud and energetic, and above all just really good fun. Along with a couple of friends, I got to know the guys who ran it. They were older students. With their studies becoming serious, they were looking for people they could trust to hand the event on to. They chose us to promote the event, sell tickets and help manage things on the night.

As club promoters, it's fair to say that we started out knowing nothing. We brought plenty of enthusiasm and untested ideas, but absolutely no experience. As a result, our learning curve was practically vertical. The main pressure was to maintain the established success of the night by keeping both the club owners and the party-goers happy. This was no small challenge for a polite, middle-class kid from the south, but it was clear that my friends and I were in it to make some good money to fund our student lifestyle. It was all good practice in negotiation and client relationships. I wanted to do the best job that I could and keep the event's reputation as one of Leeds' top nights out. Years of playing sport had taught me that, in order to make progress, you have to show up. We brought commitment to the project, and that included a willingness to learn so that, in the end, we could perform to the best of our abilities.

Securing the venue for another season was just the start. From hiring DJs to sorting ticket sales, hyping up the event, building a community and delivering a great night for everyone, we found ourselves working harder than ever. There was no rule book. This wasn't the kind of job that came with a line manager I could turn to for guidance and advice. We had to find our own way, learn from our mistakes and pledge to put on a club night that people would remember for all the right reasons.

Every Thursday night, we opened the doors to an increasing number of people. At its height, the place was rammed with hundreds of people partying. The buzz was unbelievable and, though it felt like work, I loved every moment. We were learning on the job, and our enthusiasm went a long way to making it a success. We took nothing for granted, our aim only to stage a fantastic event, and the ticket sales reflected that. In the year before we passed the responsibility on to the next generation of student club promoters, it became the most popular night on the scene. We saw upwards of 1,000 people attending, and that included the occasional celebrity, such as Harry Styles.

The experience we picked up along the way was invaluable. It wasn't something I could learn from textbooks or in a lecture theatre, but it gave me so much insight into how to get on in life. If I started out as a negotiator who was wet behind the ears, for example, I soon learned how to deal with the club's management so as to be sure I secured a fair outcome for everyone involved. That meant bringing an air of confidence to the table, but not one that could spill into arrogance. I quickly realised this came down to being polite at all times, a willingness to be flexible and creative in our discussions but firm when it came to our bottom line. If I showed respect to the people I was dealing with, they paid me back in kind, and that's how we got things done. Yes, we made mistakes and I'm sure our profit margins could have been higher. What mattered to me, though, was that we staged a great night that went from strength to strength, along with our growing insights into business.

At the time, the whole party scene was spilling from clubs to houses. I found myself at several events in student rentals that spilled out onto the street. They were great fun, but chaotic compared to our events. I shared a huge house with several of my friends who helped to host the club night. It was a Victorian terrace with spacious rooms on several levels. When someone suggested it would make the perfect venue for a club-like experience, none of us could shake the idea from our heads.

The plan was to ask for a small contribution on the door and then stage a kind of supercharged house party. We weren't doing it to get rich. We just wanted to fund the kind of quality night that we'd love ourselves. With a year's experience hosting club events under our belts, it meant we could put the plan into action. Of course, we found ourselves faced with very different challenges. First, we had to clear the house of all the furniture and contents. It took a day, and a lot of calling in favours from friends who lived nearby to take our junk and store it for us. It was hard work, but once the place was cleared, we could all see the potential.

Our plan was to stage a party for every season. We wanted to theme each one accordingly, and set up a DJ, sound and lighting system in each room. It was hugely ambitious, but in some ways we knew what we were letting ourselves in for. Pulling together, we managed to transform our student house in time for a party that we hoped people would talk about for a long time afterwards.

When 300 students showed up for our first night, it felt like our year as club promoters was effectively an apprenticeship. Without that, I would have freaked out at the number. Instead, we'd hired security on the door who also served as safety officers. Yes, it was stressful, and I imagine we would have been shut down had the police been patrolling, but somehow we pulled it off. As word spread about what a great night it had been, we all felt the pressure to make sure that the next party was bigger and better.

Things got so crazy and inventive that, for our summer party, we filled the basement with sand and staged a beach volleyball competition. It was ridiculous, and demanded so much hard work to set up and then clear away so that not a single grain was left, but it was worth it. Every party we staged proved to me that I could never just do things by half measures. That came from my experience in competitive sports, where you couldn't just phone in a performance without letting everyone down. When people are relying on you, you had to deliver to a high standard. Sure, we could have just thrown open the doors and hoped for the best, but people came to expect more than that from us, which is why they gathered in such numbers. We were putting on top-tier house parties, but for me it was all about the experience. We didn't do it as a business venture. We were students trying to have a good time and just being both creative and ambitious in how we achieved it.

Our house parties were about investing passion, heart and soul into a venture that was as enjoyable for us as it was for everyone else. I loved seeing people unite in having a good time. Whatever was going on in their worlds, they came together under our roof to let go and become a part of something bigger. I had no idea that this would become central to my work in years to come, but it was a vital introduction to skills I still call upon to this day.

The parties might have been wild, but thankfully, when it came to my studies, I kept my head throughout this time. I was at university to work towards a degree. That was always my number one priority, and it proved to be no easy task. In order to stay on top of things, I had to put in long hours of study, but I enjoyed the experience. It began to feel like the final part of a long journey to the career of my choice.

As a student, living away from home for the first time, my entire university experience taught me more about myself than I could have imagined. Everything from stretching out the student loan to make ends meet to forging friendships, sharing a house and balancing my studies with everything else that was going on in my world gave me lasting skills for life. The experience didn't shine from start to finish. I faced testing times like anyone else. Managing my workload was never easy and sometimes I'd feel stressed. It wasn't uncommon. What mattered was how I learned to deal with it constructively, which is why physical fitness continued to play such a huge role for me. I had long since come to terms with the fact that it was no longer going to lead me on the path to becoming a professional player. Instead, playing sport for pure enjoyment became an effective means of taking care of my mental health in a way that was fun and fulfilling.

I was happy, settled and loving my involvement in the city nightlife. Still, I was always mindful that, even with a degree, I would join a pool of hopefuls who shared my ambitions but had graduated from their first choice of university. As those institutions were often considered more favourably by City employers, I needed to do something to level the playing field. So, if I was going to compete for a job with shining stars from the likes of Oxford, Cambridge, Durham and Bristol, I had to make sure that my CV truly sang. In sport, when I had my sights set on a professional career in football, I learned the hard way that I could not afford to simply coast. Playing sport to a high level throughout my school years was a massive commitment and, ultimately, one that didn't work out for me in terms of becoming a professional. Even so, it taught me that, if I wanted something badly, then I needed to be able to look back knowing I had done my very best. With a City career in mind, this meant making the most of the opportunities available to me as a student. Quite simply, I was really keen to build on my degree course by getting as much hands-on experience as possible. So, when I learned about the student investment and trading society, I saw it as a potential step towards my dream goal that could also be lots of fun.

The club was just a social, informal set-up, and the idea behind it very simple. We were poor students, not professional traders, and yet we could simulate buying and selling real stocks, bonds and commodities as if we were the genuine article. The club had an online share-dealing account. This provided real-time data from the stock market, and allowed us to research, monitor, buy and sell from a pretend fund. We couldn't make actual profits or losses, and yet we took it very seriously. Together with a friend, Seb, we read up on companies, assessed their prospects and then assembled what we hoped to be a strong and dynamic portfolio.

By trading virtually, my aim was to get my head around how the market worked without risking real money. I had learned all about the mechanics of the trading floor on my degree course, but it was only when I joined the investment and trading society that I realised there could be no substitute for this kind of hands-on experience. I found it fascinating. Together with Seb, I started devoting much of my spare time to analysing the market. My dyslexia meant I still struggled with reading, and so this simulated trading provided a new, exciting way for me to learn. The virtual money felt very real to me. I didn't invest with any sense of recklessness. I learned how to assess degrees of risk and ways to balance the fund as if it were a ship at sea. I came to understand that, even if the financial wind blew in my favour, I should be ready in case a storm rose up without warning. I made mistakes, of course, but that was all part of the learning process. Crucially, it gave me a huge respect for the art of trading without the risk of losing everything in the process.

As well as hosting events for members to understand different aspects of trading, the society was one of many university societies to hold events in which speakers from different industries would come in and talk to us. One such event was a *Dragons' Den*-style pitching competition, with several guests acting as judges emulating the likes of Peter Jones and Deborah Meaden. It was fun, but also a chance to understand what entrepreneurs faced in getting a business venture off the ground.

I absorbed as much information as I could. Seb and I were so involved that one year we even put our names forward to join the committee at the club's AGM. As all the students on the board were standing down, it fell to us to take up the running to keep it going. We had no idea what we were doing, but Seb and I really loved that club. We didn't want to see it just fade away.

In the same way that I had thrown myself wholeheartedly into staging the club night and the house parties, I set out, this time with Seb's help, to do the same thing with the investment society. We really wanted to make it a success and draw in students who shared our enthusiasm. As a result, Seb and I decided to put ambition at the forefront of the society. We were committed to growing our virtual fund, and set about marketing and promoting the society as if it was a club night. We managed to attract 100s of new members, and that created a buzz about our plans. When we had enough members on board, we set about delegating tasks to volunteers. We appointed heads of sectors, such as pharmaceuticals and biotechnology, mining, tech and real estate. In turn, they recruited analysts (a fancy name for more club members) to drill into each sector for insight so as to build a strategy, then collectively we pooled our findings and steered a course.

Just as our virtual fund began to tick along, the society received an offer of sponsorship that raised the stakes considerably. We'd struck up a relationship with a local investment firm. They were experienced in the field and we had basically set out to draw on their knowledge, wisdom and insight. What we didn't expect from them was a £10,000 gift for the club to invest in the stock market for real. To a bunch of students, this was a huge amount of money and an opportunity we couldn't turn down, especially as there was no catch. Team members from the firm had started out as we had and they were just looking to inspire the next generation (and no doubt hire any shining stars). It meant that if we made a loss then we would learn from the experience, while any gains could be invested back into the society.

As a win–win opportunity, we could not wait to get stuck in. As word spread that we had real backing, so more students began to sign up as society members; keen to get stuck in with us. Seb and I went from being the only two people at the AGM to being at the heart of a popular, thriving outfit. Having picked up valuable insight into trading with our virtual fund, however, we also knew to treat the stock market with a huge amount of respect. None of us wanted to report back that we had made a loss, and that was a real driver for everyone in the society to pull together.

With real money to invest, we started holding weekly meetings for our sector heads. They pitched their investment ideas to the group and collectively we devised a strategy. In every way, we were simulating the management of a big fund. The sense of responsibility and camaraderie that created was incredible, and I learned so much in the process.

It all came down to due diligence. Those who put in the work made better informed decisions, which, in turn, allowed them to make money. I also recognised the power of delegation. Rather than become an expert in mining, for example, I learned to trust the judgement of those individuals we chose to represent us in that space. Having set out with a view to learn about the stock market, I came away having acquired wider skills in terms of teamwork. Collectively, I can only think we made every move with such care and attention that we minimised our risks considerably. Why? Because in that financial year we made gains. Finding ourselves 7 per cent up on our initial investment, we folded the profit into the society.

That moment was so exciting for us all. We had worked incredibly hard to make our student fund a success, and learned a great deal in the process. There was just so much passion swirling around a society that had been all but dead one year earlier. For me, it was a chance to put everything I had learned in the lecture hall into practice. That revealed a whole new level of practical understanding to me. In one sense we were completely winging it, but over time that experience shaped our skill sets. It gave me insight and understanding I could never have gleaned from books, and that would work in my favour when it came to entering the finance market. We were an amateur society and yet, in our year of trading, we effectively put ourselves through an invaluable apprenticeship.

*

THE VALUE OF EXPERIENCE

We can define ourselves in all sorts of different ways, from our profession to our passions, our family or social tribe. If we were to find a way to bring these components together, we can say that each and every one of us is the sum total of our experience. This is what shapes us over time, but we don't need to think of ourselves as passengers on this journey. We can play an active role in extracting the most out of our formative experiences in order to play to our strengths.

We could be talking about fleeting moments that make a lasting impression upon us, from a first kiss to learning of the loss of a loved one, to long-term episodes in our lives such as our school years, a first job or an awakening and commitment to fitness. We are all unique; our experiences reflect that.

In order to make further sense of a concept that can seem overwhelming, let's think about experiences as either planned or unplanned events. A great deal of our lives are effectively scheduled. We grow up, get educated and enter the adult world. Within this sphere, we can choose to follow certain paths. I devoted a great deal of my early years to sport, for example, and then chose subjects through school that would support a career in finance. I had control over these experiences in order to pick up certain skills and pursue a desired outcome. At the same time, a vast amount of our experiences are shaped by circumstance. Looking at life in this way, we can say that every day is a learning opportunity. We have varying amounts of control over these kinds of events, but that doesn't make them any less vital than those we choose to embrace.

I wanted to learn to become a good striker. I opted to spend time in front of the goal my dad and I built in our back garden, and there I just practised to sharpen my skills. I had no such designs to become a public speaker, however. It wasn't a lifelong ambition. My mother gave me no option but to join my sisters at drama classes because I was too young to stay at home alone. I didn't love the lessons. I would rather have spent that time on my free kicks. It felt like a waste of my time back then. As it turned out, that time on stage would prove to be a vital introduction to performing on a public platform, which forms the backbone of my life today.

In building from experience, let's begin by looking back at our lives in terms of the formative moments we went through not just by design but also circumstance. This allows us to broaden our horizons beyond the skills we set out to pick up. Ultimately, everything we do in life can work to our advantage, even if we're unaware of it at the time.

OPEN YOUR MIND

Had I dug in my heels and refused to join my sisters at drama class, my life would have taken a different path, I'm sure of it. Despite my reluctance to stand on stage – frankly, the singing mortified me – it proved to be a grounding that would serve me well throughout the years. I could call upon the experience before my first time speaking in front of a school assembly. It didn't stop me from feeling terrified at the prospect of addressing a packed hall, but it was probably enough to stop me from throwing a sickie. From there, I started to build my communication skills. It didn't come easily, but I realised that, if I wanted to get on in life, then it was a useful tool. Now, if I look back at the boy who edged onto that stage and compare him to where I am today, I realise that journey proved transformative. Had I resisted my mum's insistence that I attend that class, it could have failed to launch at all.

We all have stories like this. By just pausing for thought, we can quickly begin to count the unplanned experiences that have served us so well. While we can't undo the past and revisit opportunities we resisted, it can inform our mindset looking forward. In short, we owe it to ourselves to be open to new experiences. At the same time, we're often put off because they take us out of our comfort zones. Whether it's public speaking, parachuting or ballroom dancing, it's common for us to feel as if we don't have what it takes. The irony is that experience is the only way to build the skills we need to get to grips with the unfamiliar and even shine. That means going through a process where we have to start from scratch. It's about having faith in ourselves and recognising that practice and commitment will deliver results. Even if it's a work in progress that lasts for years, every attempt is a step forwards.

Mine and my friends' first go at hosting a club night was shaky at best. It was just something I fell into with friends. We wanted it to be a success, however, and were quick to learn from each event. There was never a time when I could say that I had cracked it, but that was part of the challenge and the reward. I was constantly learning new skills, many of which were transferable. I'm no longer in a world in which I need to deal frequently with nightclub owners, but it schooled me in the art of negotiation. I'm still on the learning curve, but with the steepest part of the climb behind me I'm free to refine and finesse the basics to suit new situations. Looking back, it would have been easy to call it quits after our first event. It took time and effort to reach a standard as club promoters where we could be proud of our achievements. We made missteps and mistakes, but we learned from them. Ultimately that experienced shaped me, and I wouldn't change it for the world.

We can all open our minds to new experiences. By recognising the barriers and learning to overcome them – from a fear of the unknown to feeling that somehow it's not part of the game plan – we give ourselves the opportunity to explore new pathways.

LEARNING FROM OUR EXPERIENCES

The cautionary experience

Over the course of a lifetime, we interact with countless individuals. There are many in this number who we like, respect and admire, from friends and family, to mentors and even people we consider to be heroes. Our interactions with them shape us. Often, our most memorable moments are those we share with others.

Then there are those encounters with people who don't chime with our values. These still have value in terms of life learning. For one thing, if we only interacted with individuals who shared our outlook and interests, the world would be a dull place. The same can be said for bad experiences. In a very effective way, it's the things we dislike that inform our values. These are the lessons that can hold true value, even if it feels like a negative experience at the time.

When I first started thinking about following my dad into a finance career, he was kind enough to bring me to work with him. It was an opportunity to see behind the trading scenes and proved to be quite a wake-up call. I had gone in expecting it to be a scene of high-stakes drama, only to discover I didn't quite chime with the bullish atmosphere. While I came away feeling rattled because it had punctured my dream, it highlighted an aspect of my character that would help me to make informed decisions. I didn't want to be that trader yelling 'BUY!' and 'SELL!' down two phone lines. I was interested in working with people on a deeper, more considered level, and that work experience sealed that deal for me.

We can all think of people or places that didn't sit comfortably with our values. I only had a brief exposure to bullies at school, who picked me out because I was physically different from them and dyslexic, but that unpleasant experience was enough for me to register that I never wanted to behave like that. If anything, it encouraged me to be more sensitive towards people who feel sidelined or excluded. This further underpinned my decision to spend less time playing team sports at university – where the alpha energy seemed more focused on drinking than winning – and that decision ultimately led me to a love of the gym.

Sometimes, though, an experience or encounter with someone doesn't have to be negative to highlight that it's not what we want in our lives. It can just flag up that something is missing that we need. I grew up in a comfortable commuter-belt town. It suited my parents down to the ground, but, over time, I came to realise that I wanted more dynamism from my surroundings. Without that background, I wouldn't have set my sights on a life in the capital.

When it comes to any kind of experience or individual behaviour, what matters is how we respond. We can fall into bad ways, for example, because it's easier than taking a stand, but where does that take us? In order to become the best version of ourselves, let's make informed decisions about how it shapes our values. This way, experience of every stripe can only become a growing force for good as we seek to make the most of our lives. Incredible change happens when we decide to take control of the controllables.

The experiences we need

We know there are skills, knowledge and value to be had from planned and unplanned experiences, including those that shine a light on how we don't want to be. That leaves just one other form of experience for us to consider, and that's the kind we *need*. It might not be something we strongly like or dislike, but one that serves a means to an end. As I worked towards a career in finance, I realised that I had a lack of experience and understanding of spreadsheet management and analytics. It hardly set my world on fire with excitement, but I took the time to teach myself. It gave me a new skill set and, by extension, that helped me in the workplace. In short, it qualified me to get ahead.

Not all the experiences we need involve a workshop, a course or – in my case – hours spent watching YouTube tutorials. Often, it comes down to refining or amplifying basic social skills. Communication is a case in point. As a teenager, I was good at mumbling at my parents but I knew that wouldn't wash when the catering business hired me to serve food at events. With tips in the mix, I realised very quickly that I needed to be polite, warm and friendly with everyone. I had to overcome any sense of shyness and just be bold. It took me out of my comfort zone, but as I built on the experience, it became easier. At the time, it wasn't a skill that I longed to master, but it brought me good tips and, more importantly, perhaps, it has served me well in all areas of my life. In finding the confidence to be sociable and engage with people around me, I discovered an improved version of myself.

So, how do we identify the skills we need? We're talking about areas that don't necessarily appeal to our interests, after all. The key is to be switched on to our surroundings, honest with ourselves about our abilities and prepared to adapt. In finding myself running an investment society at university, I realised that I needed to get organised and learn to delegate. In some ways, it was a formative introduction to being in a position of authority. This wasn't something I had ever dreamed of doing. At the same time, I wanted the society to be a success. The most effective way to achieve that, I realised, was by embracing the experience and learning on the job. In picking up the experience we need in this way, along with planned and unplanned experience, we can fill our toolkit with a suite of skills for every situation. It builds in a dynamism and flexibility that we wouldn't find by simply focusing on formal training.

PLAYING TO OUR ADVANTAGE – STRENGTHS AND LIMITATIONS

I used to be a firm believer in the concept that we should focus on turning our weaknesses into strengths. It's an admirable view, and encourages us to grapple with a challenging skill or pursuit until we've mastered it. There are many times, in fact, when this approach will reap rewards. It encourages us to overcome hurdles, and that's an outlook which can only serve us well through life.

As I grow older, however, I have come to recognise that there is also value in recognising our limitations and focusing on areas that allow us to shine. I appreciate it's an unconventional view, but I prefer to think of it as flexible thinking that we can call upon in certain situations. I only have to think of my experience as a triathlete to feel confident that it's an approach that has worked for me. I am a strong runner and cyclist, but the third discipline in the sport has always been my weakness. As a swimmer, I am average at best. I have worked to improve my stroke and speed, but in competition, I struggle to keep up with the pack.

Eventually, I reached a point where I had to recognise my limitations. The effort I was making to become a better swimmer just wasn't delivering results. It was then I decided that my time would be better spent doubling down on training as a runner and rider. That was where I was continuing to make the most improvements, after all. Having reached a point in the water where I was passable, I just focused my attention on the disciplines where I could make a difference. It was an approach that delivered results and worked for me on that occasion. The key, I believe, is to be realistic. I have no doubt there will be times when immersing myself in a specific experience will turn a weak skill into a strength, but I aim to keep an open mind for those occasions when I just need to get by so I can shine elsewhere. In reaching that decision, the question we can each ask ourselves is: what is important to us here? That is the key when it comes not just to performance but enjoyment of the experience, and I believe that both are interlocked.

It was my dad who first set this train of thought in my mind when my hopes of becoming a professional footballer fell away. Did I want to excel at the game, he asked, and sacrifice everything else in order to try to earn the right to be a professional footballer? Or did I want to play all the sports I loved and just bring sunshine into my life? As a concept, there is no wrong or right answer here. It's purely subjective. What matters is that our answer comes from the heart. And in my case it did.

RIDING THE LEARNING CURVE

We know that a first experience in a new field can be daunting. We're in unfamiliar territory and need to acquire new skills in order to progress. Our attitude is key here as it determines how we'll perform. While a fear of failure can sometimes persuade people to avoid the challenge altogether, others falter when an early experience proves uncomfortably testing.

In order to overcome this hurdle, we need to visualise our place on the learning curve. What might be difficult to begin can quickly become much easier with experience, such as riding a bike or speaking in public. With experience, that tough phase can quickly pass. Some people thrive here, in fact, because the improvements can be notable as they get up to speed. It's when that line of growth begins to flatten, however, and the rewards become fewer and farther between, that some find the real challenge begins. From there, in order to rise to the top of our game, we don't just need the basic skills from experience, but commitment, focus and determination in order to refine them.

This is the moment on the curve that really interests me. It's so rewarding for me as a coach to see people ride the steep slope of experience and gather skills and confidence on the journey. It's when that performance levels off, however, that we need to make a decision. Are we in pursuit of excellence here or are we content with the basic skills acquired? Often, those skills open up opportunities elsewhere, which is another factor in the mix as we work towards an answer. As a student club promoter, for example, I was comfortable pushing ticket sales every week to fill the venue. However, I had no desire to become the most formidable haggler in the city and squeeze every last penny out of a deal. I just set out to reach a point where I could be fair and respectful because that led to a rewarding working relationship. Crucially, it freed me up to focus on all the other disciplines I needed to work on in order to stage a successful event. So, let's pick our skills from experience with an ultimate goal in mind, and ask ourselves just how far we need to ride the learning curve for each one to get to where we want to be.

THE SUM OF OUR EXPERIENCES

Let's take a look at that moment when we run into someone we haven't seen for ages. Maybe it's an old school friend. Years have passed since we last hung out. Despite being close back in the day, and reminiscing about the same memories, it can seem like we're strangers to each other. Why? Because from the moment we followed different paths through life, our respective experiences shaped us into who we are today. It just goes to show what a powerful impact the external world can have on our values, outlook and character.

We know that most experiences are beyond our control, but we can still govern how we respond to them, and that should align with our values. Our experiences also most certainly shape us, but we can have a hand in the final design. It all comes back to thinking smart and checking in with ourselves on a regular basis. This may even extend to resetting and rebuilding to be sure we're in the best possible shape to pursue our goals. We only have to look at any top-flight football team to see this approach in action. They'll face hard games and easy games in a season, as well as matches that defy prediction. What matters is that they're match fit at any time in order to meet the challenge and are focused on progressing through the league in pursuit of both excellence and opportunity.

We can also be time-pressed, which is why priorities are important. It means picking off the experiences that serve a purpose (from pleasure to professional reasons) and identifying just how far we want to take it. Do we want to enjoy a weekly 5K with friends, for example, or train to run a marathon in search of a PB? Both experiences might start at the same place, and with equally rewarding outcomes, but the commitment and discipline involved in fulfilling those goals differ wildly. Asking ourselves that simple question before we take on a new experience is the surest way to avoid drift and disappointment, and ultimately instil purpose in our lives.

RAISE THE BAR: MILESTONES

- Our experience is determined by circumstance or design. Both are equally valuable. Your present circumstances don't determine where you can go, they merely determine where you start. Your circumstances don't define you, your decisions going forward do.
- Past experiences are building blocks for the future. Even negative episodes can become learning opportunities to help us thrive.
- Focusing on experiences we need can help us to overcome weaknesses and turn them into strengths, such as learning to be confident in social situations.

PART 3

RESISTANCE

We often consider challenges and even failures to be unfortunate. In raising the bar, I want us to think of them as vital learning moments that promote growth.

CHAPTER 5

FROM REJECTION TO RESILIENCE

Resilience is a tool for life that supports
our ambitions and drive for growth.

Leeds was a different world compared to where I had grown up. This was my chance to live an independent life and expand my horizons in new ways. It also sparked a wanderlust in me. I had always loved listening to stories from my grandfather about his exploits in different continents and countries, but my focus was on graduating with a degree that would open doors in the City.

Like me, plenty of university students with hopes of a career in finance sought internships during the holidays. It was a chance to pick up experience which might make a CV shine, while forging contacts useful in future. Critically, many positions also paid a wage. I figured if I could land work that earned me some money then I could take time out for the last few weeks before the new term started to head overseas. I had plenty of friends who shared my outlook. So, we hatched a plan to find employment wherever we could and then regroup with our passports, sunglasses and board shorts. After my first year at university, I completed an internship at an investment bank, shadowing various teams, which gave me more of an insight into the world of finance. While it was interesting and a chance to get financial experience under my belt, I also needed to try other things to figure out if it was for me in the long term. However, with a decent sum to fund the remaining weeks before the new term, my friends and I toured across Cambodia and South-east Asia. It was an incredible experience, and I returned absolutely set on leaning into the challenges and opportunities that travel had presented me with.

During my second year, I applied for a summer internship that reflected my revised career ambitions. Having decided that the trading floor might not be for me, I found myself drawn towards management consultancy. This involved working with companies to ensure they functioned efficiently. It demanded analytical skills and long-term planning, both of which really appealed to me.

Throughout my second year at university, it really felt like everything was coming together. I was enjoying my course. I was working hard at my studies, and still playing football and rugby on a regular basis. I also had a wide circle of friends, many of whom came from running the student club, house parties and my involvement in the investment society. I was happy, focused and committed to making the most of my life as a student. I had no idea that, after the summer break, all of that would seem far removed from where I found myself.

A placement year is a chance for students to continue their studies overseas. At Leeds, this meant taking a year out to focus on a specialist subject relating to a degree back home, and then returning to complete one's studies. Thanks to a network of universities around the world that were affiliated to the programme, it had proven to be a popular scheme on my course, although I came to the idea quite late. If I'm honest, I was dating a student on my course at the time and she had seized the opportunity and the only way that I could keep the relationship afloat, I decided, was by taking a year out myself so that we would return to Leeds to complete our fourth and final year together. So, I looked through the courses that still had spaces and settled on one to study international business and finance. It was split into two six-month modules. I would spend one half of the year in Shanghai and the next in Paris, which sounded great.

Then, just before we flew out to begin our 12 months apart, my girlfriend broke up with me.

It was the last thing I wanted to see happen, and the first of many testing times I would face in the year overseas that followed. First and foremost, I found the culture shock in Shanghai to be far more intense than I had imagined. I was a long way from home, far away from my friends, and my knowledge of Mandarin Chinese was practically non-existent. I was excited to be studying in China, but as the weeks and months ticked by, it felt more like a front I was trying to maintain for my own sake. I was not just heartbroken but also badly homesick.

As much as I wanted to be the international traveller, I felt isolated in a country where the language barrier made it so hard to carry out everyday tasks. Everything from buying food to catching a bus and even getting a haircut proved to be quite stressful and complicated. I couldn't take anything for granted and that made it hard to relax.

Life inside the business school was equally tough for me. It was a

French business school with a campus in Shanghai, so the vast majority of students were native French speakers. I found myself compelled to communicate in another language that didn't come naturally. It was tough to make good friends in a city that seemed to me to revolve around cliques, and I found myself living quite an isolated existence. Ultimately, the reality of living so far away didn't match up with the expectation, nor my experiences of travelling over the summer before. I couldn't help feeling that I should have stayed at Leeds, completed my degree and then set about climbing my career ladder. Instead, I was living in a flat in a vast apartment block with a sense that I had taken a year-long diversion at a time when I should have been pushing for the finish line. I regretted letting a relationship without much foundation lead me into this situation, but I also took responsibility for it. I saw it as a life lesson and took some comfort in the fact that, in future, my decisions would come from the head, as much as the heart.

Mentally, it was tough, however. While I kept up with my work, I lost the drive that had carried me through school and university. It was as if I had switched to autopilot. I did everything that was expected of me on the course, but I just lacked the passion, and that spilled into other areas of my life. My diet took a serious downswing. It was mostly dictated by what I could buy, and often by the fact I didn't know what I was even eating. Team sports – usually the tonic to keeping me sane – were out of the question, however. The language barrier prevented me from finding out what was on offer and then communicating my desire to get involved. As a result, my fitness began to decline. It left me feeling flat and, though I was determined not to waste my time in China, I never truly felt like I spread my wings. The isolation forced me to dig deep, and I began to look forward to the day that I relocated to Paris to complete the course. I didn't realise it at the time, but when I left Shanghai behind, I was pretty depressed.

In my mind, I believed that six months in Paris would be a chance to breathe. It was closer to home, after all, and easier for me to fit into the European way of life. In many ways, it proved to be a lot less stressful. Everything from greeting people to crossing roads wasn't something I had to think twice about. I also had friends who had been studying in the French capital for the whole year. They were happily settled, but also practically fluent in the language. For me, both in and out of college, I quickly came to realise that my basic grasp of French would not be enough to help me settle in that easily. In trying my best to buy a pint of milk or order a coffee, I found that Parisians just weren't willing to comprehend what I was saying. Unless I was word perfect, they'd just look at me as if I was talking Martian. Sometimes the shutters would come down so hard on my attempts to communicate that people would just refuse to continue. Back in Leeds, I used to run a successful club night. In Paris, I often struggled to even gain entry.

I found the experience incredibly frustrating. At any other time of my life, I would have been able to brush it off. Coming as it did after six months of feeling like I'd been living on another planet, my resolve was not as strong as it might normally have been. I wasn't sleeping or eating that well and, while I kept my studies ticking over, I felt anxious and generally unhappy.

Which is why I decided it was time to get fit again.

I had grown up living a highly active life. Feeling in good shape was second nature to me. I never put much conscious effort into it. I just trained and played a lot of sport. From the moment I left the UK to study overseas for a year, I had let my physical health slide and my mental health followed. At the time, I didn't make a conscious connection between the two. I just realised that I missed that feel-good emotion that came from playing games like football and rugby. I couldn't bring myself to start looking for teams in Paris that might take me on. My confidence had taken too much of a blow. I'd also run out of patience when it came to the effort I was required to make in order to communicate on a basic level. With this in mind, a session in the gym seemed like the best and most simple solution. I wouldn't have to talk or rely on other people. I could just tune out and do my own thing.

The gym closest to my accommodation block was small and basic, but with good vibes. From my first solitary session, and every day throughout my time in Paris onwards, that little back room became my sanctuary – much like our members now, many of whom have created a sanctuary that houses their Peloton equipment. I didn't need to speak a language to work out on my own, and it was blissful. I felt good, physically and mentally, and that helped me to shine in other areas of my life. I made more of an effort with my diet. I slept better and that allowed me to improve my focus on my studies. My confidence returned and that led to me making the most of my social life. I constructed each day around a gym session, and that helped me to find myself again.

Gradually, Paris no longer felt hostile. I never quite found my place in it, but I did rekindle that sense of excitement that comes from exploring new locations. Without doubt, I would have just hidden away without that chance to work out. I had been using the gym across my sporting career to improve my performance on the pitch and track, but never as the main way of keeping me fit and healthy. Nor had I ever truly appreciated the strong connection between physical and mental wellbeing. In those closing months of my year away, I learned how to best look after my mind and body. It had started from a low point, but by the time I completed the course and returned for my final year at Leeds, I felt physically and mentally stronger as an individual. I had gone through a quietly testing time but learned vital lessons from the experience. I hadn't just developed muscle from getting into shape. In terms of my resilience in the face of challenging times, I had toughened up considerably.

My placement year had taught me a lot but not being in the country for 12 months also made it challenging to land an internship that summer. Despite applying to a range of consultancy firms, I could not land a placement. Unwilling to stack shelves or loaf on the sofa at home, I decided that any work vaguely relevant to my degree had to be worthwhile, which is how I spent my internship working for a recruitment firm that focused on finding people roles within the consulting industry. It was the last thing I expected to do, but I discovered that I really enjoyed it. I had to rely on my initiative to seek out suitable candidates for vacancy shortlists, and work to strict deadlines. I was part of a team, but was expected to deliver results by running with the ball on my own terms. It wasn't easy, but I thrived on the challenge.

Above all, I found I loved working with people. It involved earning the trust of the people I was headhunting. I had something to offer them, but to do so I had to build a working relationship with them first so they recognised we were on the same side. It was rewarding in lots of ways when a candidate secured a position. It felt like a real achievement, and a buzz to help those people make decisions that ultimately benefited their welfare. There was also commission to be made on top of my basic salary. By the time the internship came to an end, I left confident that I didn't want a career crunching numbers. That element of human interaction was important to me.

My final year at Leeds University felt like I was preparing to face the world. It was as if I had brought a sense of maturity back with me from China and France, and that helped me to stay focused. Rather than unwinding by going out to club nights, I spent time playing football with friends or working out at the university gym. It struck me as a far more positive activity, and one I had genuinely grown to love. At the same time, the old competitive spirit in me remained as strong as ever. Many of my friends who hadn't taken a year out to study abroad had now graduated. Some had done so with flying colours and landed dream jobs. I couldn't help but interpret that as pressure on me, which weighed heavily on my shoulders when it came to my final exams.

I was old enough to take responsibility for my own mind state. Learning not to measure myself against other people was something that took me some time. I just hadn't quite cracked it before I graduated, with one grade short of the First Class Honours I had been hoping for. Even with a 2:1, I couldn't look back and say that I should have worked harder. I had tried my level best and was happy with the outcome. I was just keenly aware that, in a competitive job market, I would be up against candidates who had shinier degrees than mine. It was a concern that began to take root when my job applications failed to hit their mark. I was applying for posts with leading banks and corporations, and when I started receiving knockbacks, I had to remind myself not to panic.

As if I needed to make life more challenging, I had announced to my parents that I would be moving to London. It seemed like the obvious place to be in order to start a career in the City. Rather than get on board with my plan, however, they both cast doubt by flagging up the reality of the situation.

'How are you going to support yourself?' my dad asked, and it was a good question.

The cost of living in the capital was crazy. The only way that I could realistically survive there was by finding work that paid well. This added to the stress of my job-hunting, at a time when I should have just accepted it was a challenge and worked through the process step by step.

Finally, after sending off endless applications, an opening presented itself to me that would have been the ideal first rung on the ladder in a banking career. I should have been delighted. Instead, because the job on offer was in a similar field of work as my dad, I wobbled. Having shadowed him years earlier and decided it wasn't right, I had put trading behind me. Now I had an offer for a graduate-level entry job on the fundraising side and I choked.

My heart just wasn't in it, whereas my interest had grown in other areas of the industry. My experience with the investment and trading society had really opened my eyes to how private equity firms worked with people as much as businesses to promote growth. I had really loved my short time as a headhunter because it involved building relationships. The job on offer to me was mostly about number-crunching, however. It offered everything I didn't want to do.

Before accepting the post, I decided to throw the dice and apply for a graduate scheme with a private equity firm. It was one of the few big companies that offered a programme like this. As a result, it was heavily over-subscribed. I mentioned my situation to a few friends who had graduated a year before me. They just advised me to take the job on offer as a safe bet, but that wasn't how I operated. In the short time I'd spent in recruitment consultancy, I had come to appreciate the many routes that could be taken to securing the ideal job. With this in mind, I was unwilling to walk away from at least giving the private equity firm a shot, and could barely believe my luck when I was invited to an interview.

It was a chance to pitch myself face to face with an employer at a dream company, and I seized it. After the year I'd had in China and France, feeling like I'd taken a misstep, I was all the more determined to present myself as a candidate with passion and commitment. I talked about my experience in running clubs and even house parties, and essentially sold myself to the very best of my abilities. Without doubt, those 12 months of solitude and self-doubt had strengthened my resolve. I had come through it tougher for the experience and committed to making my ambitions a reality.

I brought everything I had to that interview table. Even though I couldn't match the competition in terms of qualification or experience, it earned me a place on a shortlist for a series of specialised tests. I was assessed on my aptitude and ability in everything from analytics to economic modelling. It was tough and, at times, I had to go with instinct in the absence of experience. I just wanted to give it my best shot so that I could look back without regret. As the recruitment process reached the end, I'd survived to be one of just three candidates under consideration for two positions.

And the decision didn't go my way.

I had come so close, only to miss out in the closing stage. The news came like a hammer blow. I had invested my hopes and dreams into that opportunity. I should have been more cautious, of course, but by then it was too late. I just saw it as a ship that had sailed, and so I took the initial investments job offer because I didn't want to sink.

Maybe my head was in the wrong place, because after just a matter of days working in my new role, I was deeply unhappy. It seemed like all my misgivings about the role played out. It struck me as a very bullish environment for men who like to consider themselves as alphas. It was the kind of atmosphere that sometimes took over rugby squads. As much as I liked to be a team player, I had never got on with that kind of full-on machismo and banter that, based on past experience, was basically disguised bullying.

In my first week, I was invited out with colleagues for lunch. It seemed like a good way to meet everyone, I thought, until I realised that we weren't stepping into a restaurant but a strip club. I just couldn't believe this kind of thing still happened. It wasn't the kind of energy I wanted to be around. Back at the office, I just focused on doing a decent job so I didn't attract attention to myself for the wrong reasons. It felt like the kind of place where anyone who failed to perform to expectation was considered a weak link. I had no plans to give in. All I could do was hope that a passion for the job might grow over time. What I hadn't banked on was a miracle two weeks after I started work. It took the form of a phone call from the private equity firm with the graduate scheme.

'The other candidate has had to pull out,' one of the team members who had been part of the selection process informed me. 'If you're still available, Ben, we'd like to offer you the position.'

By then, I had committed to the job I was doing at the time. I'd signed a contract that felt like a sentence, and yet I understood that it served to protect me as much as the firm. Still, I couldn't just walk away from this glimmer of hope. So, I went to see my boss. I figured in this situation I needed to be both respectful and honest with him. We'd only known each other for a short time, but we got along well. I knew that I wasn't coming to him with the best news, but he understood. As I hadn't yet worked through my probation period, beyond which I would have been tied in to the job, he suggested I could use that as my exit route. I was so glad that I'd stepped up to ask, and also was very grateful to him for giving me this out.

Two days later, I began my training programme with the private equity firm. Not in the London offices, where I would be based, but at the company's global headquarters in Philadelphia. I'd had to fly out to the States at short notice because the programme had just started and my employers wanted me there as soon as I could get on a plane. There, I joined graduates from a host of different countries who had gathered for an intensive schooling in long-term investment strategies. It proved to be the polar opposite of the job I had just left behind. Rather than living off adrenalin as we cooked up quick deals, we were encouraged to think and make informed decisions. Despite the shock of suddenly finding myself in a different role on the other side of the Atlantic, I felt so much more at home with the work and the people around me.

I was only 22 and one of the younger graduates on the scheme. I had my own small apartment in the city and, with no language barrier in play, I didn't feel cut off in any way. I was used to starting out in new cities, but this time I felt genuine excitement. It felt like I had landed on my feet, but it became clear quickly that I was among a very smart cohort of intakes – that if I wanted to prove myself, and stop feeling like an imposter, I would have to put in all the hours that I could find.

By then, a session in the gym had become one of the foundations of my day. I needed time to work out and clear my head, reset and prepare myself to go again with what I considered to be the job of a lifetime. As the reality set in, however, and it became apparent to me that I had so much to learn in order to perform this role, I found myself relying on that exercise time just to stay grounded. There was no way that I could allow myself to fall short. Having come so far, not just in terms of the miles but the time and energy I had spent dreaming of a career like this, I saw no other option.

I spent just over eight weeks training in Philadelphia. When I flew home, ready to begin work at the London office, I returned with a basic understanding of the complex skill set I would need to sharpen if I wanted to be successful in my job. I was also completely exhausted.

WHAT IS RESILIENCE?

To me, resilience is a mental muscle. It's a form of inner strength that allows us to face a challenging situation constructively. All too often, however, we fall into thinking of resilience in physical terms. A pumped physique might be the result of punishing workouts, but it's what's on the inside that really counts, and that's invisible to the eye.

Some of the strongest people I have met in my life weren't cut out to lift heavy weights until their eyeballs bulged. I'm talking about people who have faced serious illnesses with a smile or setbacks in their lives that could have persuaded many others just to give up. That's what resilience means to me. It's a quality we can choose to embrace without visiting a gym – we can even grow from the experience of overcoming obstacles that might first seem beyond our reach.

Resilience does not guarantee success. At least not straight away. If anything, that mental toughness is born from finding ourselves far from our comfort zones. For me, resilience comes from moments in our lives when it feels like things aren't going our way. Often, it's not a pleasant experience. Sometimes, it can seem crushing. When the opportunities to be a part of a professional football academy started slipping away, it broke my heart. Living alone in China, feeling cut off from my friends and family as much as the world around me, I faced moments in which I just wanted to curl up into a ball. Factor in all those times when I almost failed to make the cut, from schools to university and my first steps into a finance career, and by rights I should be used to veering off course. What kept me on track is that quality that we all have the potential to unleash – resilience.

Every single one of us can look back at our lives to date and count the bumps along the way. Very few of us have had a smooth ride, and those who pin all their hopes on out-and-out success often pay a price further down the line when things don't work out so effortlessly. We often consider challenges and even failures to be unfortunate. In raising the bar, I want us to think of them as vital learning moments that promote growth.

We all face difficult times in our personal and professional lives. They might not always be welcome, but in every case, they shine a light on who we are. Do we run away from the issue or find a way to deal with it? The answer comes back to our values, because this is when they're tested. Do we have what it takes to repair a friendship, stand up and speak in front of an audience or climb a mountain of every kind? Resilience isn't just about courage, it manifests itself as a combination of both physical and mental strength. It's about understanding our abilities, knowing where to find support and gain skills or experience if we need it, and recognising that failing doesn't have to be final. Ultimately, it can be the start of a fulfilling journey that transforms us on every level.

So, let's set aside the outdated image of resilience, which often views failure as a weakness, and explore what it really takes to be tough. I believe resilience is a quality that's available to everyone, whatever their background, age or experience; it can become the tool that builds both confidence and ambition moving forwards. Often, it comes down to a willingness to learn and acquire new skills. Even if they don't seem relevant at the time, they can only help us to feel match fit for all eventualities.

BORN TOUGH?

We tend to think of babies as fragile, vulnerable humans who rely on our protection for survival. This is true in many ways, but so is the fact that they're also hard as nails. When hungry, in need of winding or a nappy change, babies tend not to keep quiet and hope for the best. They'll cry for attention and wind up the drama to deafening levels. That takes effort in the face of uncertainty. It also earns rewards.

Later in their development, when they learn to walk, they'll spend more time flat on their face than on their feet. For all the falls, however, they persist in putting one foot in front of the other until they've mastered the art. From what I've been told, it's an incredible thing to witness as a parent. We often don't realise we've played a key role in helping our child build resilience. It's our encouragement, support and modelling behaviours that push our offspring on to keep trying. As we'll see, this is a key part of the process when it comes to taking on new challenges. When help is combined with courage and determination, plus a willingness to pick ourselves up and learn from experiences, resilience is a formidable force. Given that we rely on it from the moment we arrive in this world, it's something we just need to acknowledge and awaken within ourselves rather than learn from scratch.

THE ROAD TO RESILIENCE

We can argue that resilience is linked to an instinct for survival, but it's also something we can grow through experience. It isn't just a question of repeatedly tackling a challenge until we luck out. True resilience requires us to adapt to a difficult situation. This might mean recognising our weaknesses and turning them into strengths, relying on teamwork, training or advice to help us through, or simply thinking creatively as we plan and prepare to try again. It also means recognising that failing is not a source of shame or embarrassment. With the right outlook, it's a learning opportunity.

I started playing football from a very early age. What began as a means of channelling the energies of an overactive little boy quickly became a passion for me. I loved to play, and I loved to win, but I didn't like losing at all. To be honest, who does? But, thanks to my dad, I didn't brood about it for too long. Instead, he'd help me to work out how I could improve as a team player, so that, when I played again, I could step up my contribution.

As much as I played to win, there was nothing I liked more than being the one who scored. I wanted to be the best player on the pitch, but that didn't come served on a plate. I had to train hard, not just with the junior team I played for, but at home in our back garden. Over time, and having put in the effort, I became the player known for scoring goals. It was also the moment when I had to learn to be resilient. Why? Because all I had done was shine as a player in a little league. It would have been easy to just stay at that level and keep putting the ball into the back of the net. It would also have lacked any challenge. It meant, if I wanted to keep improving, then I had to move up to a team in the next league, and that meant starting from scratch.

As a little boy, it was tough to go from being the best player in one team to the weakest link in the next. As I had set such high expectations for myself, however, I also knew what needed to be done, and so the process began all over again. It took time, effort, hard work and the tireless support of my father. His touchline manner left me mortified at times, but it also fuelled my determination to improve just to silence him. All these components came together to build that mental core we call resilience. It takes time to establish, and the more we learn that challenges exist to be overcome, the stronger it grows.

I believe resilience is a constant work in progress. Even with my background in sport, I found that studying abroad for a year tested me in new ways. I hadn't banked on feeling so isolated and adrift, but without doubt my time on both the football and rugby pitch, as well as the running track, taught me that I could find ways to get through it. In the same way, in seeking to kick-start my finance career I was gutted to fall at the final hurdle of the graduate selection process. It really hurt, and yet that's a natural response to rejection. Whenever it seemed like I was missing out in life, I learned that I had to pick myself up if I wanted another chance. That's what drove me to seek out another opportunity and make the most of it. Had I conceded defeat and just stayed at home, I doubt I would have been reconsidered for the graduate scheme when their initial choice let them down. At every step of the way, a growing resilience ensured that I never gave up on making the most of my life.

Even today, as a coach on a high-profile platform, I'm faced with new experiences that take me out of my comfort zone. Media appearances are a case in point, but I don't let my nerves get the better of me. I've learned over time that, with preparation and determination, I can face them head on. Even if I come away feeling like I could have done better, it's a learning experience for next time. I've even started to relax and enjoy being in front of the camera or microphone, and that's something I intend to build upon. For me, resilience is a tool for life that supports our ambitions and drive for growth. As long as we're smart in taking on new challenges, it can only grow stronger throughout the course of our lives.

SHOWING UP FOR YOURSELF

What limits us in life? Can we put a name to the brake that is often applied within us when we face a difficult task or testing time? In almost every case, it comes down to a fear of failure. This could be triggered by anything from a lack of self-belief or unwillingness to risk being seen as anything other than a winner. As soon as it creeps into the equation, however, it can undermine our resolve and persuade us not to try.

We live in a world in which we've been conditioned to think that failure is a mark of shame or embarrassment. The way I see it, failure is part of the process on the road to success. It's the mountain that stands before us and the finish line, and we owe it to ourselves to rethink the reason for its existence. Is it there to stop us in our tracks and remind us of our limitations? Or does it serve to test our true character as we strive to overcome it and reveal qualities about ourselves we didn't know we possessed?

As a trainer, I find there is joy in helping clients face seemingly impossible challenges. It's a privilege to help someone find their feet and build the skills and confidence they need to go from being a beginner to meeting their goals. They start with self-doubt and then replace that with self-belief. It's like being present when the stabilisers come off the bike. I'm there to provide a steadying hand before finally letting them go. And on every occasion, they never look back. From learning to ride, applying for a new job or setting out to run a marathon, we all face mountains in our lives, but it's only by reaching each new level that we can set our sights on new horizons.

One way to see that mountain in a positive light is to consider our approach to climbing it. We could have a go to the point of exhaustion, slide back down and go again with diminishing chances of success. If this were our only option, understandably most of us wouldn't go much further than the first attempt. This is a shame because failure is effectively the first step on a journey of personal growth. It's about accepting the challenge that the task is hard, and then finding ways to maximise your chances of success. In order to summit, however, we have to show up at the foot of that mountain in the first place. It takes courage to place ourselves in that position, far from our comfort zone, and that comes from bringing the resilience we need to recognise that setbacks along the way are opportunities to come back stronger.

RESILIENCE UNBOXED

We've recognised the role that resilience can play in helping us to aim high. Now let's look at the four factors that feed into this core human quality available to us all. Just be aware that we're all unique. When it comes to resilience, each of us assembles the building blocks we have in different ways. We only have to look at the various ways in which professional athletes strive to perform at optimum levels. There is no single way to train for a boxing match or tennis tournament. Everyone calls upon common factors, which combine to form what we call resilience, but how you do so to unleash your full potential is entirely your call. Let's look at each one in turn.

RESILIENCE – FINDING YOUR COMMON FACTORS

Be self-aware

When we've set our sights on an objective, one that can seem just beyond our reach, it's very easy to compare our attempts to others and feel we're falling short. It's a sure-fire way to insecurity and doubt, which is the last thing we need when it comes to performing at our level best.

To be frank, we tend to be very good at paying attention to how other people are performing. How often have you looked over in a workout class to see what the person next to you is doing? If we just switch the focus on to our own efforts, under a searching but constructive light, immediately we are only in competition with ourselves. It doesn't guarantee we'll be best in class every time, but it gives us every opportunity to meet – or even exceed – our own expectations.

When it comes to building our resilience, we need to be switched on to how we're performing. That doesn't mean patting ourselves on the back when things are going well or beating ourselves up when they don't. It's simply about running a constant systems check and knowing how to act in order to maintain that focus on achieving our goals. When my ultimate aim of becoming a professional footballer started to fade away, I had to review whether football should be my career ambition or something I played for fun while I devoted my efforts to study. I made a decision to opt for the latter, based on that experience, and it proved to be the making of me and my relationship with sport. In China, I lost that 'systems check' internal dialogue to a certain extent. It was only in Paris, when I found purpose at the gym, that I came to appreciate the importance of constantly checking in with myself.

We all have moments in our lives when we reflect on our aims and objectives. In every case, the best outcome arises from making informed decisions. We only have to think of the data-driven reviews that take place at top-level sport to appreciate that knowledge is power when it comes to self-improvement.

We're talking about thinking smart here, whether or not we have gadgets or technical tools to support it, and that begins with a level of honesty that can sometimes feel uncomfortable. Here, it's vital that we make realistic assessments about ourselves and our abilities. I know that I will never come close to Usain Bolt's 100-metre world record time (and, mostly, people will draw the same conclusion about themselves). If I refused to recognise this fact, however, I'd only face disappointment every time I sprung out of the blocks. But what if I accept that his record is safe from my grasp, and instead set realistic targets for myself? Even if they're just beyond my reach, that keeps me incentivised, giving me something to aim for, allowing me to train to become the best sprinter I can be.

Self-awareness doesn't just allow us to think smart and adapt our approach to any challenge to maximise the chance of success, it also enables us to train smart. So, if we fail, we can assess what went wrong and learn from our mistakes. It also means knowing when to ask for help, support and advice when we need it, which brings us to the next component in our resilience toolkit.

Pick a team

Even when we pursue a goal alone, chances are we rely on information and advice to support our efforts. The internet is a treasure trove in this respect, and it's only natural that we equip ourselves with as much knowledge as we can about the challenge we face as part of our preparation. In the same way, we can increase our chances of success by assembling people around us who can get behind what we're doing. We do exactly that when we're unwell, by checking in with a doctor, or when it comes to buying a house, working with an estate agent. These are experts in their field, and we can apply the same approach to our health and fitness – whether it's a personal trainer to help you with your workouts, a nutritionist to help you with your diet or perhaps a therapist to help you with your mental health. It's important to build a team of people or team of resources you can tap into to guide you in the right direction.

As well as practical or technical advice, it's important that we can count on people around us for emotional support when we need it. Depending on the nature of the challenge, anyone from friends to family could prove to be crucial. Whether they're cheering from the sidelines, crunching the numbers to determine if we're on course for a PB or providing a shoulder to cry on if we miss out by a second, our resilience is fuelled by a network of support we can trust.

Everyone has different demands, of course, but it all comes down to a simple question: who can help me when I need it? Growing up, I was fortunate enough to have my dad at my side. He encouraged me to keep pushing, refusing to let me tread water. On those car journeys home from a football match, even if we'd won, he'd focus on an aspect of my game in which I could have done better. As much as it seemed harsh at the time, I am in no doubt that my dad laid the foundations for my drive and I will always be grateful to him for that. He was my mentor, my critic, my coach and my friend all rolled into one. Most importantly, I trusted my dad's advice.

Who we choose to listen to should form a key part of assembling our support network. It can change from goal to goal, of course, and be as formal or as relaxed as we see fit. What matters, however, is that every person believes in us and what we're doing. There is no room for naysayers, who cast doubt on our dreams or ambitions. It's vital that our team has our backs. Not only does that mean we'll get the best out of them – from encouragement to wisdom to constructive criticism and insight – but we can also be secure in the knowledge that we're not alone as we strive to reach that summit.

Bouncing back from failure

Nobody likes to fail. We set out to achieve, but if we're at the limit of our abilities, there is a good chance that success lies beyond our reach. It's not how far you fall, but how high you bounce back that counts. If we've been committed in our preparations, it's only natural to be left disappointed or even devastated when things don't work out. If anything, it's a sign that we care. When I was applying to hundreds of different internships and jobs throughout my time at university, it hit me hard when the rejection emails would come through. However, I realised quickly that most of the time these rejections were nothing to do with how much I was putting into the application, but simply automatic, based on criteria the company had set, and that was out of my control. Every failed application was a new opportunity to learn more about the interview process and more about how to show up as the best version of myself. All too often, we see people fail and then become diminished by the experience. Rather than take ownership of what's happened, it becomes a source of shame or even regret for them.

There is no such thing as failure in my life, just experiences and reactions to them. Every new experience is a learning opportunity and even if it doesn't feel great to not arrive where you had set out to go, you are wiser, more experienced and more skilled than when you started. We are all building our dream life, brick by brick and each new experience gives you more bricks and materials to build another part of that life.

It's also worth reminding ourselves that there's no rush here. Some people can bounce back from disappointment very quickly, while others need time and space. The key is that we're tuned into how we're feeling and acknowledge that help and support are always available. Treat the bounce-back phase as if recovering from physical injury. By giving ourselves time to heal, we can be sure that we're in the best possible shape, whatever we choose to do next. It can only set us up for another shot at the goal that escaped us the first time – or allow us to fully invest our energies elsewhere.

Setting goals

At the start of every year, many of us like to set new goals for the year ahead. Setting goals is an incredibly powerful tool to keep ourselves accountable in taking actions towards building the life we want to live. However, have we been getting the process of setting goals wrong all along? Many of us start this process by defining the end goal (the WHAT) and using this as our motivation. We could pledge to quit smoking or drinking, set out to become the top scorer in a football team or harbour ambitions to become world-famous in our field. Whether our vision is concerned with our personal lives or set to change the world, we're talking about the target that we set out to reach. Ever since I was a young boy, I have dreamed of being able to support a happy and healthy family. I want to be an amazing partner and father, and live a life filled with joy and fulfilment. For me, that is the ultimate driver in everything I do.

Personally, before determining WHAT I want to accomplish, I thrive on the concept of taking the time to find the WHY. The purpose, cause or belief behind a goal will be the thing that motivates me to overcome the inevitable hard times along the way. It's the very reason the goal exists in the first place and the compelling higher purpose that inspires me and acts as the source of all that I do. I want to be able to support a happy and healthy family because that is where I see myself gaining the most joy in my life going forward. I am passionate about leaving a legacy behind me and this goal will allow me to do this. Our goals need to feel good. And those feel-good goals come from giving voice to your WHY. When you hit on the values and emotions that drive why you want to achieve a goal, a light goes on in the brain and kicks your body into action.

The next step in my process is to understand the 'HOW'. The process and specific actions I'm going to take to realise the WHY for that goal. I like to use vision boards to build and refine that picture, because that's just how I'm wired, and I also like to build small goals and review time into this process. Why? Because if we're talking about a ten-year plan, for example, then age, changing circumstances and needs all come into play. It's one thing to pursue a dream, but not if we outgrow it or even discover it's making us miserable. That driving passion must be at the core of everything we do, and if it's not there we owe it to ourselves to regroup and redefine where we're heading. You may have heard of SMART goals: Specific, Measurable, Achievable, Relevant, Time-Bound. Once you have your why and your vision, it's time to employ this method for both your long- and short-term goals.

It's important to give yourself permission to change course. Too often, we set ourselves grand and adventurous goals and refuse to bend the rules. There will be job opportunities and life opportunities that we can't even imagine right now in the future for us all. Understanding our WHY, HOW and WHAT will allow us to keep ourselves 'match fit' for when those opportunities arise. Establishing a destination, with a route map for the journey, is the surest way to instil purpose in everything we do.

RESILIENCE FOR LIFE

We've seen the role this strong inner core can play in helping us to raise the bar. We know that it's a quality that we call upon from a very early age, and which we can strengthen with experience over time. Resilience is an incredible resource, available to us all, and not least because it can be applied to all manner of different situations. It's a transferable skill.

I learned about knockbacks at a very early age. It wasn't a pleasant feeling to find myself left out of a football squad. With support from my dad, I just had to recognise that it was an opportunity for me to find out what the coach needed to see from me in order to get picked, then work on delivering it. That same sense of determination returned during my time studying abroad. I figured I could either wallow in feeling cut off and miserable or aim to make the most of the experience despite being limited by my grasp of another language. Even missing out on the graduate scheme on my first attempt ignited that same response in me, and I can trace it all the way back to being a kid with no place on a team. That taught me to take ownership of difficult situations, dig deep and find ways to overcome whatever stood in my way.

For me, resilience is like a superpower I can call upon when I need it. The wonderful thing is that it exists within us all, in the form of skills combined with experience, and the more we can learn to harness its potential, the further we will go.

RAISE THE BAR: MILESTONES

- Resilience is a muscle of the mind. It's a form of inner strength that allows us to face a challenging situation constructively.
- We're not born tough. Resilience grows from experiences, including those that don't go to plan.
- Don't be held back by a fear of failure. These are learning opportunities that are humbling yet bring wisdom, determination and self-belief.

CHAPTER 6

OVERCOMING OBSTACLES

No journey is without challenges.
What defines us is how we overcome them.

Through the eyes of family and friends, I was living the dream. I'd landed a sought-after job in the City. Selected as one of only two graduates in the UK for the scheme, I had a career path mapped out in front of me. My starting salary was pretty reasonable. It meant I could afford a decent flatshare in London, which proved to my parents that their son could live an independent life at last.

I should have been feeling so positive and energised about my future. Instead, I became increasingly anxious and strung out. Why? Because it quickly became apparent to me that I was faced with projects beyond my abilities. Despite all the aptitude tests, I struggled to get on top of what I was supposed to be doing. My dyslexia didn't help matters and, though I had learned coping strategies, my confidence took a knock. Rather than grasp the role and use it to maximise a return for the company, I just spent the whole time hoping people wouldn't realise

I was still grappling with the basics. It left me feeling like a blagger. It was as if I had something to hide, which meant I was on edge the whole time. Compared to my colleagues, it just seemed like all my efforts were devoted to appearing to know what I was doing rather than actually getting the job done. I started taking work home with me in order to keep up. Eventually, even the time I ring-fenced for the gym – something that had become non-negotiable for my mental wellbeing – had to go. Quite simply, my job demanded every waking hour that I had so my bosses didn't feel like they'd made a mistake in selecting me for the graduate scheme.

I was working with a colleague who had the same position as me. She was also in training, and we got along well. While she had a flare for figures and a confidently analytical mind that had earned her a science degree, I was more comfortable than her with talking to clients and building relationships. I didn't want to let her know the full extent of how challenging I found my role, but she worked it out for herself. So, we started to lean on each other a little. I would be on the phone while she was dealing with projections, and that helped each of us to get by. She was more capable than me, however. Despite her support, I still found myself working from the moment I woke up to late into the evenings. Often, I would stay up until 2am, getting to grips with a project while fuelling myself on takeaway meals and caffeine. Then, all over again, I would be first in the office, not for the sake of appearances but because I couldn't afford to fall behind.

Within a short space of time, my boss asked me how I was coping.

'Fine,' I said, a little too quickly to be convincing.

'Ben, you look exhausted,' was his response.

There was no hiding the fact that I was struggling. It was reflected in my work. I was delivering everything expected of me. It's just I was taking far longer than everyone else, and that was unsustainable. I felt like I was treading water and out of my depth, and in what felt like an alien environment, that I just didn't feel like I could ask for help. Rather than reach out and admit I needed support as I wasn't coping when my boss asked, I simply doubled down on my work in the hope that somehow I would get up to the same speed as everyone else. As a result of pretending everything was fine, I simply invited concern and even incredulity from my seniors when I took so long to complete work that should have taken half the time.

As the months ticked by, and I devoted every waking hour to my job, my work did begin to improve, however. There was no dramatic upswing in my productivity and value to the firm, but it was just enough to avoid earning too much attention at work for all the wrong reasons.

As well as the challenge I faced in getting to grips with my role, I also found it hard to fall in with the working atmosphere. At my first job, the one I had bailed from to join this firm, it had been clear to me right from the start that the *old boys' club* attitude to women and money was not for me. The episode with the lunchtime visit to the strip club had summed it up. I didn't want to play a part in that culture. While that kind of thing didn't happen in my new place of work, it shared the same bullish atmosphere towards exceeding targets and the pursuit of profit before personal welfare. This wasn't exclusive to the firm, I realised. It was ingrained across the finance industry. I had always known it existed, of course. I just hoped that

I would be able to find my place in it without having to adopt the same values.

Rather than seek to rise above it and be my own person, I was so worn down by the experience that I fell into the same mindset. I was in a job that paid very well and yet I found myself thinking about bonuses. It seemed to me that everyone around me measured themselves by how much they were earning or by their job title. It was just a driver for greed, but at the time it seemed like the established goal that everyone chased. What's more, in my line of work, many of my peers were investing their own money in business start-ups and ventures that could provide a medium- to long-term return, which is where the serious financial gains could be found. Some of them were making eye-watering amounts of money, yet I wasn't even close to possessing the kind of seed fund they were putting in to get things started. Rather than step back and ask if this was really the life I wanted to get into, I continued to hope that working myself to the bone would eventually lead to some uptick in my fortunes. Frankly, it was madness. Compared to the sports-mad kid at school, and the student hoping to go places at university, I barely recognised myself.

Throughout this time, my personal life was paying a heavy price. I functioned on very little sleep. I'd often wake up feeling more exhausted than when I went to bed. My diet was dictated by whatever takeaway I could have delivered to my door. I barely used my kitchen for anything other than making coffee or just stacking food boxes, beer and wine bottles for the recycling bin. Frankly, I didn't have time to shop for food let alone cook anything from scratch. When my gym membership expired, I let it lapse. I should have been gutted, but instead I just felt

numb and resigned to the fact that my life was different now. I knew
plenty of people who were building their careers in London, but I had
even less time available in the week to see friends. Unlike me, they
seemed so happy and forward-thinking. They also knew how to make
the most of their free time. I'd often agree to go out, only to cancel
when a wave of work threatened to crash over me. As a result, as I was
just so flaky and unpredictable, people drifted away. As for dating, my
inability to commit to anything but work made it impossible.

Operating at full tilt, I craved some form of release every now
and then. I was in such a destructive cycle, however, that rather than
wind down and recharge, I took to partying hard on a Friday and
Saturday night. I saw it as a chance to catch up with those mates who
did put up with me. I managed to hide what was going on in my life
from them and, in turn, they considered me to be this City whizz-
kid with the money and lifestyle to match. I was so tired that it just
seemed easier to live up to that stereotype, and I really went for it.
I'd show up at parties straight from the office in my suit because that
was now who I was trying to be. It was as if the role and the image
that came with it was what defined me, forgetting about all the things
that made me happy and that came before.

Drinking to excess at the weekends became the default way for me
to escape from work. Office hours had become meaningless to me
and this seemed to be the only way I could forget about the fact that
spreadsheets, projects and deadlines had come to dominate my life.
All too often, in a heaving bar or club, I'd lose track of the people I was
supposed to be with. Instead, I'd find myself hanging out with complete
strangers, and then heading home in such a mess that any recovery time

was spent hungover. It was a spectacularly self-destructive pattern of behaviour, and one that reflected my unhappiness. I was 23 years old and scared that I had trapped myself in a career that was draining the life out of me. Worst of all, I had arrived at this point by my own decision-making process. Nobody had forced me to follow this path. I felt so desperate as I only had myself to blame. With no choice, it seemed to me, but to press on blindly, I just used what time out I could scrape together as a coping mechanism.

I was burning out. There was no way that I could sustain the intensity either at work or play. At the time, however, I had just resigned myself to the fact that I was in trouble but with no escape. Frankly, all my energy went into holding down my job. When it came to looking after myself, from my personal welfare to any attempt to make changes for the better, I had nothing left. Physically, I felt terrible. I had gone from being really fit to just feeling so lethargic and out of shape. Sport had been so important to me. Since I started work, however, it had become something I caught on the TV with the sound down if I was working out of hours at home, rather than something I took part in. I was constantly on edge because I worried that somehow I'd be found out. I still felt like a fraud, despite working so hard, and that further undermined my confidence. In effect, I had entered into a declining spiral. I wasn't aware of the strain it had placed on my mental health, but it was apparent to those who knew me. When I visited my parents, their questions about how things were going contained a note of concern. I was quick to head them off from the truth, and they didn't push it, but effectively I was just deceiving myself.

Nobody is superhuman, but I considered myself to be tough. For that to be a positive force, personal welfare has to come into the mix. I was sacrificing everything for my job, while in my personal life I was dealing with grief – my beloved grandfather had just passed away. That my job was proving to be so demanding had left me painfully aware that my family time had fallen away. Finally, it reached a point where one minor issue sparked a crisis.

I made a small mistake at work. It wasn't much, just a small screw-up in a financial presentation, but after working late over four consecutive nights, it proved to be the final straw. It was my boss who picked me up on the error. I drew breath to cover for myself, as I had on many previous occasions, only for my throat to catch.

'I can't,' I blurted out, and immediately began to blink back tears. 'I can't do this any more.'

It was a moment of honesty that came as a relief. I told him that I was struggling with the spreadsheets and all the complex data-crunching, and admitted things hadn't worked out as I had hoped. I had tried my best, I said, but just didn't have anything more to give in order to meet his expectations. By then, I was beyond caring about the consequences. I assumed my boss would just tell me to pack my bags. In my short experience in the finance industry, there seemed to me to be no room for faltering or failure. I was broken. It was over. Frankly, I was feeling so destroyed that a dismissal would have been fine.

My boss just looked at me awkwardly, which was no surprise as I had started blubbing.

'Ben, you're only human,' he said. 'We'll sort this. Just pull yourself together, eh?'

As a response, it took me completely by surprise. I left the office that evening feeling both deeply relieved to have opened up but also in despair. It seemed to me that my grand plan – one I'd hatched as a young boy in awe of his father and the career he had forged – lay in ruins. I was approaching my mid-twenties, and I felt like I had made a mess of my whole life. It was not a good feeling in any shape or form.

The next morning, my boss summoned me for a chat. I hadn't got much sleep, but I'd found some composure. I had no intention of bringing emotion into the conversation again. I was just going to spare him any further hassle and quit there and then. Before I could inform him of my resignation, however, he shared a proposal that left me momentarily lost for words. My meltdown really had brought out his compassionate side, because, in the short time available to him, he'd spoken to a colleague who worked on a side of the business more involved with clients than crunching numbers. As a result, he had created an opportunity for me to move across to a position that would allow me to play to my strengths.

It was the kindest gesture that had ever been shown to me since I started my career in finance. Rather than boot me out, my boss had pulled some strings to give me this second chance, and I seized it.

I had reached the point of burnout. Like so many people, resilience had been the quality I relied on to survive this challenging time. It's a healthy quality, but what I hadn't done was look after myself in order to stay strong. Instead, in an ever-increasing state of exhaustion, I had just told myself to push on. Eventually, I had become so weak in the face of it all that I lost all awareness that help and support was always at hand.

I was ready to walk away, only for my boss to show that he wasn't going to just give up on me. As a result, I had a chance to reinvent somewhat by moving across the company. Rather than staring at figures on a computer screen, the focus of my job involved picking up the phone and talking to clients. It would mean building presentations with them and and lining up meetings with potential investors to help raise capital for the business. It was exactly the sort of thing I had enjoyed during my internship as a headhunter. At last, I felt like I had some control over my role. It was one I could embrace and call my own. I could also be a team player by liaising not just with my colleagues but the clients who relied on me to deliver results. Most of the business I handled originated in Europe, but the rest of my team were based Stateside. That meant that the bulk of my work and meetings took place after lunch, when America started trading for the day. My boss travelled most weeks and my line manager was based in the US, so coming into the office with everyone else at nine o'clock, rather than feel I needed to be at my desk several hours earlier, became my new normal.

Within a week, it felt like a glimmer of sunshine was back in my life. I had more structure to my working days. They could still be intense when my clients woke up across the Atlantic, but that was fine by me. I was no longer having to burn the candle at both ends, which meant I had energy to devote to all the right places. I had a routine at work, which was still hard but, critically, now also manageable. Best of all, I was working more efficiently, meaning I could leave it behind when I finished each day, and bring some balance to my life. It meant I could be more mindful about eating. Even though my free time was pressed, I could at least cook some of my own meals, catch up with friends or even go out for a quick drink. I was getting more sleep and, when that routine took shape, I realised just how central rest and recharging was becoming to every aspect of a busy life.

Best of all, in waking up to make the most of each day, I found I had time before work to return to the gym.

*

WHAT NOW?

No journey is without challenges. What defines us is how we overcome them. Often, we can anticipate what's coming. They might even be the reason why we're on that path in the first place. Just look at athletes chasing medals or PBs. A challenge is hard by definition. It forces us to raise our game. It also encourages us to be courageous and resilient, and brings rewards that go beyond exam grades, promotions, medals or PBs.

An obstacle is a challenge with a different complexion. These are bumps in the road that can slow us down unexpectedly. An obstacle can also be a barrier that stops us in our tracks. It can present difficulties or problems that we didn't anticipate, give rise to self-doubt and test both our motivation and mindset. All obstacles can be handled constructively, but all too often they throw us off our game. They may even leave us questioning if we can continue.

Obstacles take all shapes and forms. They can appear when we least expect it, and sometimes seemingly out of nowhere. An injury to an athlete is a case in point. It's unplanned, unwelcome and throws a training programme into disarray. In other cases, an obstacle can creep up on us so slowly that it takes some time to register what we're facing.

When I started in the finance industry, it took me quite a while before I realised that I wasn't coping with the demands of the job. I was qualified for the role, but unprepared for the workload and sense of expectation that weighed upon me. I hadn't banked on finding myself at my desk deep into the night in order to stay afloat. As time passed, my lifestyle started to suffer. I was permanently tired and anxious, not eating properly and partying at the weekend as a misguided means of escape.

The fact that I was relatively young proved to be a double-edged sword. While it meant that I could exist on little sleep, a poor diet and a great deal of stress, it just extended my misery. It also crept up on me so slowly that I became that frog in a saucepan of water; unaware of the rising temperature as it approached boiling point. It simply wasn't sustainable. Rather than deal with the situation constructively, however, I allowed it to consume me. Eventually, unable to maintain the illusion that I was coping, I broke down in front of my boss.

Looking back, it was a masterclass in how not to face an obstacle in my path.

Across the course of almost two years, there were so many subtle warning signs that I chose to ignore. Rather than take proactive steps to sort things, I just pressed on and hoped in vain that it would all become easier. In a sense, I froze. Now, I consider that testing time to be a learning experience.

OVERCOMING OBSTACLES

In facing any kind of obstacle, no matter how traumatic or seemingly impossible to overcome, we are all equipped to make informed decisions. The tools in our kit range from the practical to the emotional, so let's get to grips with them now so we're prepared should the worst occur.

Recognise

As I experienced for myself, when things don't go to plan it's easy to avoid confronting the situation. It's human nature, in fact, to respond to an unexpected or unwelcome event with a sense of shock and even denial. We can find it hard to accept, but simply ignoring the obstacle in our path won't make it go away. In every case we need a plan of action, and that begins with recognising what stands in our way. You can't fix what you can't face.

Whether or not we're responsible, often we can't change what's happened. Whether it's out of our hands or a lesson learned, it's vital that we accept the situation for what it is. Stewing in regret or even denial will just use up energy that we can use in more positive ways. At the same time, it's important to acknowledge any negative feelings that mark this moment of realisation. It's something we hadn't anticipated, after all, and could even be the last thing we need, and so it's normal to feel anything from disappointment to anger or anxiety. Owning that emotional response, and expressing it constructively, will provide a clear head necessary to assess the situation and plot a way forward.

Reach out

With an obstacle preventing our planned progress, this is the moment to turn to our team. Even if it seems as if we're on a solo venture, there will always be people around us who have our best interests at heart. From friends and family to colleagues or people on the same path, these are individuals who will understand what we're facing. They can provide anything from a listening ear to help, support and advice to even making an active contribution to getting us back on track.

In dealing with the obstacles in my finance career, I should have approached my boss when I began to feel them mount. Just talking would have helped me to make sense of the situation, and I may well have received the support I needed to get back on track. Instead, I bottled it up until I couldn't take the pressure any longer, confessing I wasn't coping in a way that took him by surprise. While it came as a relief to share the burden, I could have handled it better by arranging time to talk with him at an earlier opportunity. It was a lesson learned – and showed what a lifeline clear, direct and considered communication can be when faced with a seemingly impossible situation.

Revise

If we're unable to move whatever obstacle stands in our way, we need to devise a way to get around it or make changes to our quest. We're talking about adapting here, which could apply to anything from missing out on target grades or a job selection to picking up a sporting injury or facing funding issues. Just pressing on is often not the answer, as I discovered to my cost in the finance sector. Our smart move is to take stock of the situation, consider the options and make an informed decision about the most constructive and rewarding way forward. The key is to be flexible in our thinking. This may mean we have to make changes that feel momentarily unwelcome, or sacrifices that can hurt. Ultimately, it comes down to staying focused on our objective in a way that puts our welfare first as well as that of everyone in our team.

Review

In charting a revised course in order to overcome an obstacle, it's important that we pay close attention to how the new plan plays out. Pausing to assess progress allows us to make adjustments and improvements. If we've put the obstacle behind us, we may even be able to return to our original path and press on as intended. By monitoring our journey and staying flexible in our approach, we can be confident in the knowledge that we've charted the most effective course under the circumstances.

Taking steps to deal with any obstacle doesn't guarantee a successful outcome. What it will do, however, is provide us with ownership of the situation. Without a plan of action, it's easy to feel helpless. Only we can take charge of a difficult situation, from the feelings it triggers to the strategy to face it head on, and that begins by finding the positive in every moment of the journey.

OBSTACLES AS OPPORTUNITIES

Often, the most effective tool we have for dealing with a difficult situation is to change our perception of it. Nobody wants to experience a setback. It's not something we invite into our lives, because essentially it's standing in the way of our goal. It's natural to respond negatively to a setback, even if it's just by swearing out loud. Venting in this way is a constructive way to clear the air as much as our minds as we focus on the obstacle before us. Our aim now is not to let negative energy take over, after all, but actively seek a solution.

As a kid getting to grips with the world, I used to hate finding myself on the substitute's bench before a match. It was something I dreaded as a junior footballer and, though I managed to avoid it most of the time, I didn't respond well when my turn came around. It was my dad who helped me to manage these disappointing moments in a more positive spirit. He basically gave me two options. I could stew about not being picked to play and resent everyone from my teammates to the manager. Or, I could use the opportunity to make myself selectable. How? By talking to the manager and finding out where I needed to improve in order to earn my place on the pitch.

My dad's advice saw me back in the starting eleven the following weekend, but it also had a lasting impact on my attitude to setbacks. Some years later, in my last term at grammar school, I picked up an avoidable injury on the rugby pitch when a friend took me down with a dodgy tackle. He was only messing around, but it meant I missed out on the chance to play rugby in my first term at university. I'd been really looking forward to the opportunity. I also recognised that it was pointless being annoyed about the situation. My friend felt terrible about it for one thing, but more importantly, there was nothing I could do to change what had happened. What I had some control over was how I spent my recovery time.

So, instead of brooding, I decided to hit the gym and work to become stronger. In my mind, I wanted to strengthen my body so that, if I got tackled badly again, I would be looking at fewer than 12 weeks of recovery. In doing so, I enjoyed my first brief taste of the restorative powers of working out. By the time I returned to the rugby pitch, I looked back on the accident as the moment I learned to take better care of myself if I wanted to continue playing contact sports.

When it comes to finding the positive in obstacles, we can help ourselves by preparing in advance. It's about reviewing our attitude before we take on any kind of challenge and ensuring that our mindset will encourage us back on our feet should we suffer any kind of setback. It can only build character, even if we push towards our goal with no unexpected turns. And should the worst occur, we'll be ready to find ways to become stronger and wiser for the experience.

In some cases, we can inadvertently create obstacles for ourselves. If we've committed to a goal and put in the time and effort, it can be hard to accept that some barriers can be overcome if we just set our pride to one side and open our minds. In my early years as a personal trainer, I loved putting together house music playlists for my workout sessions. I'm passionate about the genre, and just figured everyone in my class would share the same enthusiasm. It was only later in my career that a fellow coach encouraged me to broaden my horizons. In order to reach the biggest possible audience, he advised me, I should embrace not just different genres but classics from decades like the eighties and nineties. Everyone has different tastes, after all, and in sticking to house music, I was limiting who would enjoy my rides.

My instinct was to reject the suggestion. It was well-intentioned, but surely everyone loves house, right? It wasn't until I paused to reflect and remove my personal interests from the equation that I recognised he'd made a strong point. And so, having swallowed my pride, I set about exploring new genres that I might have previously rejected as simply not being my thing. And it proved a revelation. From dancehall to reggae and hip-hop, summertime chart hits and vintage classics, not only did my expanded playlists connect with a wider audience, but I found myself with a new appreciation of music I had previously overlooked. While that initial realisation that I could do better hurt my ego, the rewards from being humble about it proved immeasurable. It helped me to feel comfortable with music that I had previously dismissed and taught me so much about being flexible in pursuit of personal growth. As a bonus, it was a learning experience to overcome an obstacle of my own making, which also turned out to be great fun.

A HELPING HAND

If obstacles are the unwanted cousins of challenges, which we willingly take on, both are a necessary feature of life. They encourage us to dig deep in different ways and assemble strategies to overcome them. In both cases, we often turn to our teams to help us through what can be a difficult time. It's one thing for us to know who is on hand to help us, but what if we find ourselves called upon when someone faces an obstacle in life? What is the most effective way to provide support if requested?

The answer is for us to consider the kind of help that we would like to receive ourselves. As a fitness coach, I regularly seek to help people improve their workout routines. I'm mindful that sometimes they might not even be aware that they're facing an obstacle (which could be of their own making in terms of incorrect technique, for example). The last thing I want to do is simply tell them they're doing it 'wrong'. In a class situation that could draw attention for negative reasons and leave that individual feeling embarrassed. With this in mind, I always think first about how I would respond to the advice I have in mind.

Here's how I can feel confident that I'm part of the solution and not the problem.

BE PART OF THE SOLUTION

Empathy first

When it comes to interacting with people, with a view to helping them make the most of an opportunity, it's vital that we begin by establishing a connection. I don't subscribe to the Sergeant Major School of ordering someone to put more effort into a task. For me, rewarding results happen if I can relate to them on a human level. We're talking about empathy here. Even if our backgrounds or circumstances differ wildly, this begins by placing ourselves in that person's shoes and asking ourselves how we would like to be helped or encouraged, supported or guided.

Be constructive

If someone is facing an obstacle, chances are it's testing them in some way. It can put them into an emotional state of mind, from stress and anxiety to disappointment, frustration and even anger. In every case, combining empathy with a constructive outlook is a sure-fire way to start off on the right foot. For me, this begins by flagging up that I've experienced struggles and frustrations of my own through life, not just with my physical health but also my mental wellbeing. In doing so, I'm reaching out from a place of understanding. It won't guarantee we can resolve the issue straight away, but we can face it together. When wrapped up with a constructive attitude, this approach shows we're here to help. Even if we don't have any instant fixes to overcome the obstacle, we're demonstrating that they're not alone in facing it.

Sometimes it's hard to know how to help someone dealing with a setback. If it's unclear, we can still support them emotionally while they figure out a way forward. Often, a listening ear is the most effective thing we can offer, and in talking things through that person will often find their own solution.

In a coaching situation, where the obstacle is often down to technique, I'll begin by highlighting what's going right. Then, I'll suggest that things could be even better if we attend to one aspect of their routine that's holding them back. Whatever the issue that stands in their path, I've set the focus on overcoming it, and doing so together.

Set out steps

There are times when an obstacle is apparent to everyone but the individual facing it. They can just be too close to the problem to see what's gone wrong, or unable to grasp the solution. I often see this as a coach and avoid just urging them to overcome whatever stands in their way. Instead, I seek to create a series of steps for them to follow. It can be just little reminders, but often they help the most. The aim is to create a lifeline for that person. Ultimately, it's about creating a process in order to lead to an outcome that puts the obstacle behind them.

In other instances, people confronted by an obstacle just want someone else to make it go away. As tempting as it might be, it's always more effective to encourage that individual to find their own way forward. As a team player, we can be on hand to provide the tools they need, from emotional to practical help. If they can overcome the obstacle on their own terms, they'll be all the more rewarded by the experience.

PREPARING FOR ANYTHING

There is something very satisfying in looking back on a successful undertaking in which an obstacle threatened to derail us. By reaching that goal, despite unexpected events, we've demonstrated a willingness to adapt on the fly and revise the strategy. It shows a forward-thinking attitude as well as compromise in some cases and even creativity.

At a time like this, it's tempting to think that our work is over. This would be to overlook the fact that obstacles and setbacks aren't necessarily a one-off event. Through life, they can strike out of nowhere or develop over time, which is why we should always be prepared.

I don't believe we need to be ready for the worst to occur. More often than not, obstacles and setbacks come as a complete surprise. If we could plan for them in advance then effectively they become challenges we can expect along the way. What's more, bracing ourselves for bad things to happen can cause us to make decisions and act out of fear. Instead, let's go into any challenge or journey prepared for all eventualities. It could go like a dream, become our worst nightmare or anything in between. By equipping ourselves with the tools should thing go wrong, we can take each step as it comes in the knowledge that we're ready for anything.

Imagine a group of adventurers are preparing to set off on a mountain hike in summertime. The temperature is clement and there's all but a breeze in the air. Half the group are prepared for anything. They've packed a first aid kit, a phone for emergencies, along with base-layer clothing designed to keep them warm. The other half of the group look on in bemusement. They're wearing flip-flops and shorts, in keeping with the weather conditions as they set off.

Now, as they head up into the mountains and the weather becomes unpredictable, we know where this hike is heading. Hopefully, they strike lucky and complete their journey without drama. But if the temperature drops or someone trips and suffers a scrape or worse, only one half of the group can say they're properly equipped.

Preparing for all eventualities can sound like a great deal of work, which could be off-putting for some. In reality, it simply requires good planning skills, which doesn't just apply to a day in the mountains, but to anything from the launch of a new project or business venture to a safety procedure at work or any kind of pursuit. We may never call upon them, but, as we set off, what they bring us is peace of mind.

RAISE THE BAR: MILESTONES

- Redefine challenges as opportunities for learning and growth. Obstacles on that journey may be unexpected – such as injury or missing out on a selection – but can always be overcome with practical and emotional tools.
- Turning to our teams at this time – from fellow players to coaches and work colleagues – can create a skill set with exponential potential for success.
- Learning to help and support others facing challenges and obstacles can also teach us how to prepare for all eventualities.

CHAPTER 7

EMBRACING OPPORTUNITY

When a door opens into the unknown,
not all of us step through without hesitation. Why not?

I believe there is a great deal that we can do to steer our own destiny. We can make informed decisions, review progress and seek to make any necessary changes. If I'm being completely real, we have to recognise that sheer luck can also play a big role.

My boss had given me a huge break when I finally admitted I wasn't coping. I hadn't even considered that I could move across the company. Had I requested a transfer, I imagine it would have gone down very badly. Instead, by breaking down in front of him and effectively showing him that I had hit rock bottom, he saw fit to offer me that lifeline. My new boss travelled a lot and placed a great deal of faith in me to get my work done. Freed from the feeling that someone was watching me and waiting for me to trip up, I was far more productive in this environment. And I actually started to enjoy my work.

From that single lucky break, a cascading effect seemed to wash over my life. Along with the structure that returned to my days, my outlook turned positive once more. It led me to look at my physical health and recognise that I had let it slide. The drive returned for me to get back to doing something that I loved. At last, I could see that neglecting my fitness had just contributed to that bleak period. While I had learned the value of asking for help when I needed it, I vowed to do everything that I could to avoid slipping into that trough of despair again.

At the time, boutique gyms were beginning to open up across London. These tended to be smaller than those offered by the fitness chains. They specialised in classes such as indoor cycling, yoga and high-intensity interval training. A strong feeling of community was forming within them. People were getting to know each other there and forming friendships based on a shared love of keeping fit. After such a long period in the wilderness with work, the social aspect really appealed to me. I had always enjoyed the solitude that came with working out alone, but for now I just craved company. So, I took out a rolling monthly subscription with a specialised booking app. This offered me a set number of classes at discounted rates in boutique gyms across the capital. I was broken after such a long, lonely and challenging time at work. My self-confidence had taken quite a hit. So, for my first class, I found a bike at the back and just thought I'd keep my head down.

For the next class, I was one of the first to arrive and took a bike at the front. Why? Because I was loving it! From the moment the instructor kicked off that first session, I came alive. I found myself swept up by the intensity of the session and how closely we locked into the rhythm of the soundtrack. It was so energising. I was equally struck by how hard the instructor worked to bring everyone together on the same ride. In the way she controlled the tempo as much as the energy levels in the room, it was like watching an orchestra conductor for bikes. I was entranced, inspired and just so enthused. For that short time, I set aside all thoughts about my life outside that moment. I stopped worrying about everything – from a call I needed to make at work to what I had to buy for supper on the way home. The general hum of life just ceased when I began to turn those wheels, replaced instead by a sense of pure freedom and joy.

What's more, it seemed to me that everyone in that class experienced the same thing. Afterwards, as we filed out looking hot in the face but happy, people were chatting and laughing together in a way that would have seemed odd anywhere else at seven o'clock in the morning. Had I been on the Tube to work at that time, everyone would have been in their own bubble of gloom. As I left the gym for the office, heading into the sunshine outside, it felt like that bubble had burst.

Booking via my app, I had intended to do one class a week. That quickly turned into two and then three, across different classes and with a range of teachers, and before long I was upgrading my subscription to be sure it kept up with my needs. Morning gym classes became a part of my daily routine. It was the means by which I started each day and set myself up for work. It was a great way for me to get up to speed, mentally and physically, and also meet new people. I got along just fine with my colleagues and clients, but inevitably our lives revolved around finance. All we ever talked about was work and money. Before and after each gym class, however, I found myself chatting with people across a wide age range and from all walks of life. There was also no hierarchy. It was all about personality rather than position.

Many boutique gyms were located in central London. It meant lots of people who showed up for classes worked in the creative and marketing industries that were situated around there. They were also passionate about their jobs. While I was deeply relieved to have found a position at work that I could handle, I started to realise that I lacked that same fire as some of them. At the time, it didn't feel like a critical part of my job that was missing. Even so, I was always drawn to hear about everyone else's latest projects at work as they spoke with such enthusiasm. Gradually, I found myself making really lovely friendships with people I would have never otherwise met. Quite simply, it was based on a shared recognition that fitness and looking after yourself could be central to a fulfilling existence. Even though we came from different walks of life, we all pulled together.

Group fitness wasn't a team sport like football or rugby. The way I saw things, it brought people closer together than that. Within weeks of my first session, I was showing up every day at a Kensington gym which I had come to consider to be my home venue. I worked nearby, which meant I could maximise my time working out before leaving for the office. Half a year on, rather than get hammered at clubs or parties, I spent my weekends meeting up with new friends and doing stuff that aligned with our shared interest. I got into cycling and we'd head out for long rides that finished with a healthy meal. It was a sea change from the City boy I had become. This felt much more like me.

As well as creating a new social circle with my classmates, I also started to become friendly with the other coaches. I'd ask lots of questions about their work, before changing into my suit and tie and heading into the office. Rather than thinking about tasks and strategies I needed to address through the day, I'd find myself reflecting on the structure of a particular workout or an inspiring phrase that a coach had used. Or send messages to the coaches about the latest superfoods or bio-hacking tools to try. While work was still tough for me since the move, I was much happier. I was playing to my strengths by liaising with clients, but deep down I knew that my growing interest in health and fitness was at the heart of it all.

'Ben, you're practically living in this gym. You know the staff, the boss and everyone who comes here. You never miss a class. Why don't you just teach one?' one of my coaches joked as we filed out from a session, and I laughed. But the fact was I'd attended so many of her classes that I pretty much knew how she was going to take everyone through it before we'd started. Then I exchanged a look with her that left us both wondering whether it might just be possible. The wheels started turning, in more ways than one – could it be possible? Could I teach?

I went to work that day with the idea lodged in my mind. I just couldn't shake it. Once I was back in the office and swamped by work, it seemed ridiculous. I had a decent job in the City, but if I was serious about leading a class, then I needed to qualify as a physical trainer (PT) first. Why would I want to spend my valuable free time gaining credentials that had nothing to do with my career?

It was a question I couldn't answer, but nor could I ignore it. Following another chat with my coach, who had basically promised me a Saturday slot if I was serious, I found myself coming up with more reasons why I should go for it than dismiss it. I had fallen in love with every aspect of the fitness lifestyle. I enjoyed the classes and the benefit to my physical and mental health. I had also made friendships that felt like family. Above all, I realised I was totally drawn to the transformative process we all went through. From the moment I signed up for my first class, fitness had become more than just a way to stay in shape, it had become a journey. It had changed every aspect of my life for the better. As a coach, perhaps that was something I could give back.

The training course was short but intense. Over six weeks, I attended classes and seminars every Saturday and squeezed in homework during the weekday evenings. Even though I was tired, I threw myself into it wholeheartedly. All the elements of the syllabus fascinated me, from anatomy and physiology to skills I had some background in like planning and working with clients. As the course progressed, it even struck me that my experience in and skills learned hosting club nights during my university days could come into play. I had to be self-motivated, competent in putting on a rewarding experience and able to safely manage the needs of different people so that everyone felt fulfilled. By the time I earned the basic licence that allowed me to coach, it no longer felt like an odd move for me to make. If anything, as a side hustle that I could take seriously, it seemed like a natural progression.

The gym lived up to its promise and offered me a weekend indoor cycling class once my paperwork was in order. It was just a single session to see how I would get on. By rights, I should have been quite relaxed about stepping up to do something that was essentially for fun.

I wasn't dependent on it for the money nor the career progression, and yet, in the days leading up to the session, I could think of nothing else. I just wanted to do a good job and, having been inspired and enthused by so many coaches, I set myself a high bar. That meant piecing my session together to make it fresh, upbeat and fun. I spent ages selecting a playlist to accompany the class and kept rehearsing it in my head as if preparing to deliver a speech. I left nothing to chance, and even got an early night before the class.

That morning as I headed into the studio, I was both excited and apprehensive. It seemed so weird to have gone from being a student to a teacher. I worried that anyone who knew me in the class might not take me seriously. Instead, those familiar faces who filed in showed me nothing but good wishes and support. And as the moment came to start the class, I didn't feel alone. They had my back.

'*Welcome, everyone. Let's get ready to ride—*'

I heard my voice and barely recognised it. This wasn't Ben from finance, who once avoided public speaking, but a completely different version of myself. I sounded confident and people responded by grasping their handlebars. For the first time in years, I was reminded of how I felt as a boy when I joined my sisters at singing and drama lessons. I was up on stage again in some ways. Now I just needed to deliver.

'*Are you ready, guys? We've got this . . .*'

It came as a relief to start turning the pedals. I had so much nervous energy and this was the release I had been waiting for. With the lights down low and the music pumping, I felt like I was leading a charge here. I had been so used to following instructions that it seemed as if

I had stepped outside of myself to watch this young guy like everyone else as he took the lead.

'*Hold strong . . . hold steady . . .*'

The air conditioning kept things cool. Even so, a sheen of sweat began to gloss my brow and shoulders. I was fired up by the responsibility and determined to deliver. All eyes were on me now, as if I was a preacher before a congregation. My nerves stayed with me, but now that I was moving I just used it to say focused. I was hyper-aware of my surroundings and every person in them, and first to notice when a latecomer slipped in at the back to join the session.

'*Now we're gonna switch things up—*'

I recognised his face straight away, which left me with my heart in my mouth. Without interrupting the flow of my class, Piers Morgan climbed onto a spare bike and proceeded to get up to speed. Of all the people to join my class, it had to be a celebrity, and not just any – a broadcaster completely unafraid to speak his mind. We made eye contact and, in that moment, I realised this first session could potentially make me. Or break me.

Even though that thought entered my mind, I knew there could only be one outcome.

If anything, seeing someone known for being so outspoken just persuaded me to take it up another level altogether. If anyone was going to criticise me, I needed to stay positive by knowing that I had put my heart and soul into the challenge. That way, if anyone tried to bring me down, I could rise above it.

I was nervous about what kind of feedback I might receive. While I had absolutely loved coaching a session, I was well aware that my enjoyment was far less important than the experience for the clients. They could review my class via the app, and so I braced myself for a bruising. Instead of poor ratings, however, I found my hard work had paid off. The feedback was great – and so inspiring. I was flying and made it my mission to build on the experience. When I caught up with the gym boss who had given me the chance, I no longer felt like such a wild card. In fact, she extended an invitation that made me feel like I was part of a team: if I wanted to coach on a weekly basis, the opportunity was mine for the taking. I seized it.

From that moment on, Saturdays became the high point of my week. Rather than sit at my desk all the way to Friday looking forward to a break, I couldn't wait to put the office behind me so that I could focus on my weekend job. I loved it so much that I didn't even linger on the fact that I was being paid to do it.

In those early days, I looked to other coaches and trainers for inspiration. I took note of things they did that I liked and admired. Then I sought to incorporate it all into my own routines in a way that made it my own. Slowly, as I built up confidence and experience, I put my mark on those sessions. As a coach, I created a presence that would get the attention and respect of my teammates in that room. It wasn't a question of becoming a caricature or even making one up from scratch. It was about looking at myself in the mirror in terms of my personality, and then playing to my strengths. Away from the gym, I'm not a naturally big character. I aim to be kind, loyal and respectful, as well as just good company. A friend once observed such qualities amount to a quiet dignity, and that was the aspect of my character I called upon from the saddle.

On a practical level, I realised that a great deal came down to how I projected my voice. All those forced drama lessons I'd had as a boy, which didn't seem relevant to my life at the time, suddenly became a vital foundation. I needed to communicate with clarity and confidence, in a way that brought people along with me. Ultimately, I had to bring an energy that motivated people to ride alongside me. In those early days at the gym, I was free to climb off my bike and walk among the class just to focus their attention as much as provide motivation, encouragement and even hype at the right moment. It was all about flow from the start to the finish of each class. Much of that could be shaped by the playlist, but really it was down to the coach to bring it home for everyone present. It was a learning process, but in doing so I discovered more about myself than I had ever done before.

I even found myself taking on extra roles at the gym, including some personal training. Working with clients on a one-to-one basis was something I did every day in finance. I enjoyed that aspect of my job but I adored it in this new role. I felt privileged in being able to take someone on their fitness journey. It involved setting realistic targets that motivated people to push themselves. There was something so rewarding in seeing that transformation. I brought so much enthusiasm with me that more gym users approached me about training them. Mindful to keep this aspect of my life ring-fenced from my real job, I built up a small roster of clients. I even took on a couple of celebrities, and it was lovely to discover that they were just as down to earth as anyone else. The money didn't compare to my salary in the City, but the experience meant a great deal more to me.

I had reached a point where my day job was going well. It was still challenging, but I was getting on top of the workload. By rights, I should have used my free time to unwind. Instead, I started to fill my weekends with as many classes and personal training sessions as I could. The first time it spilled out into a weekday morning before work, I figured it was a one-off. When that turned into three early-bird classes, I justified it by reminding myself that the bulk of my work with clients in America took place later in the day. Unlike in my first role with the company, I didn't need to be in at the crack of dawn. My classes started at 6am and yet I'd still be at my desk by 9am sharp. From that moment on, I would be completely in the zone as an investment analyst. My role as a personal trainer and coach did not impact on my work in finance. I could compartmentalise my two working lives just fine, especially as one of them was just a bit of fun, after all.

It took me about a year before I finally stopped kidding myself that coaching was a side hustle I could drop at any time. I had started competing in fitness competitions and signing up to marathons and other races to challenge myself. Having learned the power of branding from my days as a club promoter, I willingly took on a role as an ambassador trainer for Puma and was receiving attention from other brands to represent them. By then, it had reached the point where I felt completely fulfilled by my work at the gym. It was making me really happy and that, in turn, was reflected in my performance in the office.

Running a class first thing in the morning served to kick-start the energy I then brought to my work with finance clients. As I'd embraced rowing and strength sessions into my teaching repertoire, it also helped to get me back into good shape. Not only that, but I also stopped worrying what my colleagues thought when I opened up a healthy lunch at my desk rather than grabbing the standard, rushed, office sandwich. In effect, my role as a fitness coach had turned my life around, and that didn't go unnoticed by my boss at the investment company.

When I was first approached about coaching a class on Saturdays, I'd had to ask him for permission. As it could be classed as a second job, contractually it required his consent.

'That's fine,' he said at the time. 'Just make sure it doesn't affect your work.'

I imagine he was worried that I'd overstretch myself and end up back in that spot where I was struggling to keep up. Instead, it left me leaner, healthier, more alert and confident in leading projects and liaising with clients. The whole fitness way of life meant my diet had improved, I was sleeping well and had pretty much transformed from the burned-out case who first came to him. I played down just how much work I was doing at the gym, but because it was clearly benefitting my real job, I avoided any difficult questions. Then I arrived at a moment where I couldn't just quietly balance my two lives. If I wanted to keep climbing the career ladder in finance, I needed to start travelling overseas for work.

It was one thing maintaining a phone relationship with my American and European clients, but my boss was increasingly keen for me to start liaising with them face to face. The prospect of a transatlantic lifestyle should have been really appealing. Instead, I just worried that I would have to skip taking some classes and that might put my regular slots in jeopardy.

On the face of it, I should have been able to just drop the coaching.

However, by then, it had come to mean so much to me. Having been through such a desperate period in my first role at work, I was keenly aware that my passion for fitness was key to my wellbeing. I worried that if I dropped it then I risked building up a sense of misery along with my air miles.

As I dwelled on what seemed like quite a big life choice, I started talking things through with people I trusted. Mostly, this came down to the other coaches at the gym and long-term clients I had come to consider as friends. One of the things I loved about this side of my life was the fact that it brought me into contact with such a diverse range of individuals. Mixing with people who had different jobs, aims and ambitions really opened my eyes to the world beyond finance. Some were involved in start-ups, which fascinated me, while others were pursuing passions that rewarded them in ways that didn't result in becoming obsessed about money and bonuses. I really admired this way of living, and it persuaded me to consider becoming a full-time personal trainer.

What might have seemed unthinkable only a short time before had steadily grown to become something I couldn't just dismiss as sheer fantasy. Since starting at the gym, I had reviewed my own goals and money was no longer my top priority, and yet while I knew that I would love being a full-time personal trainer and fitness coach, I still worried that it would be a massive step down financially. I was sure I could manage, but did I really want to walk away from a career that I had set my heart on from an early age?

It was the sensible part of my character that won out over the dreamer. As much as I considered coaching to be a dream job,

I couldn't ignore the reality. Physical and mental health had come to be more important to me than financial wealth, but at the same time it didn't seem sensible to put myself in a position where I might have to worry about paying the bills in order to stay living in London. As a way forward, I decided that I should just keep my eye open for opportunities in the health and wellness space that might capitalise on my experience in finance. I was skilled in investing and fundraising, after all, and my knowledge of the fitness industry was growing daily. As my hybrid career was no secret at the gym, I would sometimes find clients approaching me for strategic advice about new ventures they were developing. I'd always happily advise them, while sounding out whether there might be scope for me to get involved.

In my mind, I'd reached a decision. In reality, nothing changed. I continued to coach at weekends and in the mornings before work, and just hoped my finance boss wouldn't ask me to take on a project in Europe or elsewhere, which would force my hand to quit the gym. Subconsciously, maybe I was preparing for the time when I'd have to call it a day there.

I was throwing myself wholeheartedly into each session as if it could be my last. I just came alive as a coach, and to see my classes full to capacity was all the reward I needed. I put my heart and soul into making sure that every moment counted for all my clients, whether they were regulars or new faces there for a specific fitness goal, or just to take them somewhere else before 'real like' kicked in. As the gym was a central London venue, I was quite used to fleeting visits by travelling business people and so, when a tanned, toned American guy showed up for one of my Sunday sessions, I figured he was in town for work. In a way, that's exactly why he'd flown in. It was only when the session finished that I discovered he had come to my class specifically to see me.

'Hey, that was great.' People were filing out when he crossed the floor to shake my hand. I'd barely had a chance to towel the sweat from my face. 'Would you join me for a coffee? I'd love to discuss an opportunity with you.'

Instinctively, as if seeking a way out, I glanced at my watch.

'Erm, well . . .'

Although he seemed very nice, as much as I loved to chat with clients as I got to know them, I just defaulted to being very British about a surprise invitation from a complete stranger. Then the guy grinned so warmly, it disarmed any reservations I may have had.

'Just give me 15 minutes of your time. It could change your life,' he continued.

When he introduced himself, his name wasn't familiar to me. Nor was the company he represented as one of their leading trainers. Cody Rigsby had chosen a quite spot in the café for us to talk. I sat facing him with the espresso he had just bought me and listened to him outline how Peloton aimed to reinvent fitness for everyone.

'—Imagine hosting a class but on a live-streamed global platform,' and that's when my ears pricked up. As Cody told me how this pioneering US outfit manufactured at-home gym equipment that could connect online to live workouts, it sounded like a vision of the future that was tailored just to me. I loved the idea that people could join leaderboards or even interact with each other, just as they could in class, but do so from bikes and treadmills within the comfort of their own homes. With a library of workouts available online, as well as live sessions hosted by trainers such as Cody, I was sold on the idea before I'd even finished my coffee.

It turned out Cody had come to London on a headhunting mission and I was deeply flattered that he'd heard I was a trainer who might fit in with his company's vision. At the time, I had a small Instagram account where I uploaded workouts and shots from the gym, but it was never intended as a serious showcase. Having spent a long while dreaming of making the switch to coaching full time, however, now it seemed I had an opportunity to turn that into a reality. And yet rather than seize it, I thanked him for his interest and politely said I would need to take a further look into it. 'I actually have a career in finance,' I told him. 'Coaching is just my hobby.'

With a shrug and a smile, Cody left me his card. 'Well, let's stay in touch. Ben, it would be great to have you on board. When I say this could well and truly change your life, I mean it.'

I had turned down the offer for good reason – I needed to do more research. It sounded amazing, but I had listened to him not as a trainer but in my role as an investor. Part of my finance job, before making any kind of commitment to a business, was to pull it apart on paper in order to assess its health and potential. So, I went home and did exactly that. With the public data available to me, I got myself up to speed on what I was dealing with here. I learned that Cody was in fact a big deal in the world of fitness training in America, while Peloton had been making waves there since 2012 when its co-founders devised the means for technology, hardware and production to bring exercise classes into the home. It really was a new concept in fitness and an exciting one, but I needed to be sure that Cody's pitch was underpinned by a solid business framework. Thanks to my job, I knew how to read the numbers. It didn't take me long to recognise that Peloton had shaken up the fitness industry and were pursuing a vision to expand the brand to a global market.

I was excited by the venture. It combined fitness with a forward-looking vision, and that bridged my two worlds. Despite Cody's enthusiasm, however, I wasn't entirely confident that I could be the right person to introduce the company to a British market. Operating from a small studio in New York, Peloton had a stable of about ten trainers. Most of them had backgrounds in dance or some kind of stage work. Looking them up online, these guys knew how to perform to camera, which was something I had never done.

During our conversation, Cody had explained that, if I was interested in coming on board, then I would need to send him a video answering a series of questions sent to showcase my personality. It meant that, while I was excited about Peloton, and thrilled that they considered me to be a good fit, I was pretty sure that I would fail at the hurdle in front of me. Still, I figured it had to be worth at least responding to the invitation and so I asked a mate who was good with cameras if he could film me coaching a class. The whole experience was entirely new to me. It reminded me of being thrown in at the deep end as a club promoter in Leeds. Back then, I didn't know what I was doing, but I went in determined to take it seriously. So, as the camera rolled, I told myself to give it 100 per cent. Even though I didn't feel like the consummate performer, it was important for me to project that. As a new experience, I found I quite enjoyed it. Thanks to my friend's efforts behind the camera, his patience as I did a few takes and his skill as an editor, I sent the finished film to Cody feeling like at least I'd been respectful to him, and to myself, in giving it my best shot.

I really didn't expect to hear back from him. The way I saw things, if I pinned my hopes on a positive response then I'd be lining myself up for disappointment. Then, shortly after sending the film to Cody, an event overtook my life that cast my entire future into question.

*

WHAT HOLDS US BACK?

When a door opens into the unknown, not all of us step through without hesitation. Why not? Because we're fitted with a natural survival instinct, and generally we don't like uncertainty. Yes, curiosity comes into the mix, but so does our comfort and safety, and if everything is good where we are, do we really want to leave it all behind?

A sense of familiarity is a precious commodity. If we're relaxed and unthreatened by our environment, it allows us to be ourselves. At the same time, that sense of security can be our undoing. Quite simply, it can discourage us from growing as individuals because we don't want to lose our comfort blankets in life. As a result, when an opportunity presents itself, many of us will turn it down for all the wrong reasons.

It's easy to regret something we haven't done. That's why this chapter is devoted to being smart when it comes to opportunity so we can make informed decisions. We're talking about an invitation to embrace something that might be new, unfamiliar or a step up from what we know. A great opportunity is always going to test us in some ways. We just need to lay the groundwork to be assured that we stand every chance of success no matter how challenging it might be. Even if we fail, we can still make it a learning experience that helps us to grow and ultimately shine.

When I think about the opportunities that have come my way, there's always one consideration that can threaten to hold me back. Like so many people, a little social anxiety is an aspect of my personality that would have restricted my life if I'd let it. Over time, I've learned to overcome it, and even feel comfortable projecting the more outgoing side of my character. Had I just given in to that temptation to stay on the quiet side, there's no way that I'd be leading the life I have today. For me, learning to build my confidence and engage with people has led to all sorts of opportunities arising. In rare cases, I have seized them without question. Others I have politely turned down because they didn't feel right for me. In most cases, when presented with a chance to do something new, interesting or challenging – and usually all three at the same time – I have taken time to do my research. This way, I can minimise the uncertainty and know that I am making the right call.

OUR APPETITE FOR RISK

During my time in finance, I learned the importance of evaluating just how much risk I was prepared to take before making an investment. All sorts of factors played into the outcome, from the financial health of the business we were looking to support to the wider state of the market in which it operated. In addition, it was important that I had a clear understanding of my appetite for risk. This became key to the whole venture. If I was uncomfortable with the commitment, that could affect my ability to make the right calls. I know that I am quite cautious by nature, which is why I didn't enjoy my work experience on the trading floor with my dad, and I am comfortable with that. We can't be judged by what level of risk we're prepared to take. We're simply talking about understanding an aspect of our character that allows us to operate to the best of our abilities.

Beyond business, our personal appetite for risk is just as important when it comes to assessing opportunity. Often, when we're presented with the chance to take on something new, that fear of the unknown holds us back. Even if it appears to be a dream come true, we're reluctant to leave our familiar environment behind just in case it proves to be a nightmare. In real terms, we could be talking about anything from accepting a job offer in an industry that's new to us to trying an unfamiliar dish on holiday. Risk is a factor in our everyday lives, and so it's worth just pausing to consider how much we're prepared to carry.

In assessing our risk, one simple question we can ask when faced with a new opportunity is 'what's the worst that can happen?' We're talking about identifying the scenario, deciding if we should make a commitment and figuring out what to do if it fails to work out. If we taste an unfamiliar food, then at the very worst it's not to our taste. With little to lose, this might encourage us to give it a try. If we're talking about moving from a salaried but unfulfilling job to one that's exciting but only pays on commission, however, we need to ask if we're comfortable with an uncertain income. If we have financial responsibilities, such as rent or a family, they will factor into our appetite for that particular opportunity.

In asking ourselves this question, each time we're faced with a chance to embrace something different, it means we have a base on which to ground our decision. Ultimately, our appetite for risk is a measure of the confidence we carry into any commitment, which is vital for everything from our happiness to success.

WHEN OPPORTUNITY KNOCKS

Over time, I've learned to respond to a new opportunity by doing my research. Whatever our appetite for risk, most of us would like to reduce any uncertainty. Shining a light on the invitation in question can only help us to see what's in store before we take things further.

Without doing our homework, we're at risk of acting on an opportunity in one of two uninformed ways. First, there's a strong chance we take it on without a clear picture of what we're facing. Think of a job interview in which we strive to say all the right things without really knowing much about the role beyond what we've read in the advert. Even if we make a good impression, we could be setting ourselves up for a fall by promising so much without being sure we can deliver. This does us no favours. If I look back at my decision to pursue a finance position on the graduate scheme post-university, I realise I could have made more effort to find out what was involved. I was so focused on being accepted that I neglected to explore some of the aspects of the role I would go on to find so difficult. Had I done so, I might have considered following my dad's approach to getting into the industry by starting low and working upwards. That way, I could have got to grips with the challenges by degree rather than being overwhelmed by them. I don't regret my move into finance. It taught me a great deal about myself as well as an industry that fascinated me. Even though I took the long road to fitness, it led me to where I am today. I also learned from experience that it's always worth making time to fully explore an opportunity before committing because ultimately that gives us options.

While it's tempting to skip the research to embrace a compelling opportunity, I am also amazed just how many people turn *down* chances because they don't know enough about them. If I was invited to do a parachute jump, I would be torn between wanting to seize the chance and my gut instinct to keep my feet on the ground where they belong. Without doing my research, there's a good chance that I would pass on the offer. If I just stopped to look into what's involved, I'd be able to make a decision based on facts and not fear. So, let's look at a three-stage approach to working out if an opportunity is the right fit for us.

THE THREE-PRONGED APPROACH

1. Due diligence

Players in the world of finance and business rest their reputations on this approach to new projects and ventures. Before entering into any kind of agreement or contract, they investigate all aspects of the proposed relationship to be sure they know what they're getting into. In short, it's a fact-finding mission. The aim is to remove or minimise risk and uncertainty, and this is something we can apply on a personal level to assessing new opportunities.

When people learn about my background in investment banking, they assume I must have taken a huge risk to become a personal trainer. They're worlds apart, without a doubt, and yet I didn't just leap from one role to the other. That would have gone beyond my appetite for risk, creating anxiety and uncertainty, which none of us need.

In reality, my transition from finance to fitness was both gradual and controlled, much of which came down to planning ahead to minimise all risk. When I first discovered a real sense of belonging and happiness at the gym, I didn't imagine that one day it might become central to my professional life. Instead, I just found myself increasingly drawn to all aspects of the industry. I enjoyed being a student in class and, when it was suggested that I should train to host one, I gave it careful consideration. In terms of due diligence, I looked into the qualification process. On establishing that it took place at weekends, outside of office hours, I saw no conflict of interest with my employment. When it came to teaching classes, however, I consulted with my boss for the sake of transparency. At no stage did I take any chances. The way I saw things, in fact, I had nothing to lose.

Later, when Cody Rigsby approached me and introduced me to Peloton, I undertook a similar evaluation process. Thanks to my background in finance and investment, I could drill into all aspects of the company to feel confident about everything from their values to their business model and strategies for the future. At the time, my passion for fitness had grown to the extent that I had a particular interest in businesses within this space. Through my eyes, Peloton were pioneers of a concept to bring the gym class into our homes that appealed directly to me. They offered something totally different, combining convenience with engagement, and by providing a safe and accessible space for people to be totally and authentically themselves.

From the comfort of their own homes, Peloton members could sing along to song lyrics at the top of their voice without anyone looking at them strangely (apart from maybe their family or pets). They could wear whatever clothes they felt comfortable to work out in, along with endless options of training types and class lengths, and choose when to work out on their own terms. This was an outfit that had cracked how to break out of the traditional gym format, and I wanted to be part of that ride. In terms of due diligence, I just ensured that my head as much as my heart was as involved in any decision I made.

2. Talk to key players

In considering any opportunity, a key part of my research is to reach out to people with experience or insight. In my view, this is the most effective way to find out more about what's involved on a human level. If I'm still debating whether or not parachuting is for me, for example, I would talk to people who have thrown themselves from great heights in the name of fun. I might even contact an instructor to find out more about the procedure and put my safety concerns to rest.

In every case, knowledge is power. We need to put some effort into finding out the facts, but the return means we can back ourselves with confidence. The more we know about an opportunity, the easier it becomes to choose if it's right for us. Just as we might decide that a parachute jump under professional guidance is in fact a safe way to seek the ultimate adrenalin hit, so we could also opt to pass on an inviting job offer because everyone we've talked to who is associated with the business has had nothing but critical things to say. At the end of the day, it's a personal decision. We just owe it to ourselves to make it enlightened.

3. Consider the timing

Had I gone straight into personal training, skipping my short finance career, I doubt I would have found much success. If I'm honest with myself, I lacked the communication skills required to carry everyone in the class with me. I needed those years working with clients whose businesses we had invested in. It taught me the value of listening and diplomacy, encouragement and sensitivity. Without these qualities, learned through experience, I would have brought enthusiasm to my coaching role and nothing more. In short, I would have been in the right job at the wrong time, severely limiting my chance to grow as a coach.

Timing is a critical factor when it comes to considering any opportunity. There are so many factors that can come into play, which boils down to individual circumstance. Among others, we need to consider where we are with our lives at that time, what commitments we have and the degree of risk involved.

Talking things through with someone we trust is an effective way to find answers to our questions, but really it comes down to a personal decision. Just be careful not to use timing as an excuse to turn down an opportunity because you lack the confidence. We have to be honest with ourselves here. Change can be scary, even if we've done our due diligence, but change is also a catalyst for growth. Yes, there could well be challenges ahead, but, essentially, we're talking about the chance to learn new skills and thrive from wider experiences.

CREATING OPPORTUNITY

People don't always come knocking at our door. If we sat around waiting for that life-changing invitation, we could find ourselves disappointed. If we're motivated, willing to learn and focused on personal growth, there is nothing to stop us reaching for our own opportunities.

From passion projects to side hustles, or even heading new ventures and businesses, the smart move is to put in the research first. By reducing the risks, talking to people with knowledge and insight to share and considering the timing, we can create new pathways in our quest.

We are no longer in an age where we stay in the same job until retirement. Today, we have to be flexible and dynamic in our approach to opportunity. In some ways, there's no greater control on offer than steering one of our own creation. Yes, there are often risks associated with going it alone, which is why we must never lose sight of the concept that we are always part of a team. From friends and family to colleagues and associates, even contacts we've made along the way, there is always someone we can count on to support us if we set out to build opportunities. What's more, by tailoring them to our values, the rewards begin from the moment we tread that new path. An opportunity of our own making might well be challenging, but isn't that what learning and growth is all about?

MAXIMISING OPPORTUNITY

We know that making considered decisions is the best way to act on opportunity. If we've made the commitment, however, it's important that we then focus our energies on maximising the moment. It isn't just about proving to the boss that they made a sound investment in us. On a personal level, it's important that we make every effort to live up to our promise and potential.

At the same time, it's worth recognising the difference between embracing an opportunity for the right reasons and being opportunistic. The latter might bring short-term gain – in the form of a pay rise, for example – but if that's the sole reason for moving on, then will it really prove to be fulfilling? We have to be smart about this at all times. We don't tend to have one shot at an opportunity in life. In some shape or form, we're presented with them all the time. What matters is that we choose them wisely, earning our chance to progress, and in a way that allows us to make a positive impact. This way, each opportunity becomes a stepping stone that allows us to advance with confidence, at our own pace, on a journey that's rewarding on so many different levels.

RAISE THE BAR: MILESTONES

- Opportunities can take us out of our comfort zones, which makes it tempting to hold back. Research, due diligence and smart thinking about our appetite for risk allow us to make an informed decision and move forward with confidence.
- Be ready to create opportunity that allows for long-term development and growth, from pursuing a passion project to a work promotion. A flexible and dynamic outlook means we're constantly moving in the right direction.
- On embracing any opportunity, aim to maximise the return. It might demand energy and commitment, but always enables us to live up to our potential.

CHAPTER 8

OUTER JEWELS VS INNER HAPPINESS

We need to revisit the concept of happiness,
recognise its value and work to place it at the heart of our lives.

'Ben, I hope you don't mind me saying this, but please can you see your GP as soon as possible?'

I had just finished coaching a class when one of my clients approached me. She looked a little awkward but also concerned. Then she told me she was a doctor.

'What's up?'

'It's just you have a lot of moles.' She now had my full attention. 'I've noticed a few that I really think you should get checked out.'

It took me a moment to process what she was saying. As everyone else had filed out of the class, I thought she was going to ask me about the timetable and not something this personal or potentially alarming about my health. I was well aware that my mole count was higher than for most people. It had never bothered me, however, and nor had I ever thought to pay close attention to them. Growing up, I had always thought it was just one of those things. Now my client was telling me that she'd had a friend who died of skin cancer. Since then, she'd taken it upon herself to urge people like me to get checked out.

'Thanks,' I said, trying hard not to sound too shocked. 'I'll do just that.'

I was true to my word because the episode rattled me. At 25 years of age, I'd never paused to think about that kind of thing. I was young. I'd only visited hospital once in my whole life, for my broken collar bone. My world was just opening up to me, and suddenly I'd been advised to get a professional medical assessment possibly for something serious that in my young mind only ever happened to other people.

I managed to get an appointment before work the next day. My client had assured me it was something to do just to be on the safe side. Having slept on it overnight, I headed in feeling a little more relaxed. I was just doing the sensible thing, so I didn't have to worry.

If I had hoped that my doctor would dispel my anxiety in one visit, I was wrong. Instead, his decision to refer me to a dermatologist strung it out for a few more days. When I got to see the skin expert, he took a biopsy, or sample, and sent it off for testing just for peace of mind. Even though he had said that the mole on my lower back looked odd, I left feeling as if the results would just be a formality. I was fit and healthy. People like me didn't get cancer. Of course, now, I see how naive I was in thinking this.

'—Ben, I'm sorry to tell you that the results have come back. The mole we were concerned about is a malignant melanoma.'

'Skin cancer?' I knew the answer before he confirmed it. I had to remind myself to breathe. 'You can just cut it out, right?'

'We can remove it, but I have to be honest, in terms of grading, you're on the borderline between stage 2 and 3. That means there is a chance it has spread from the skin to your lymph node system. We will act now, and do everything we can to fight this, but I have to tell you, without treatment this is likely to spread fast and your survival rate will start to drop dramatically if we don't move fast.'

I went numb. The dermatologist assured me that he was just outlining a worst-case scenario so that I knew what we were dealing with. Even so, it felt like I had just stared death in the face.

When I finally emerged into daylight outside the clinic, after the dermatologist had administered a local anaesthetic and removed the melanoma with a scalpel, I closed the main door behind me and burst into tears. I had gone from debating my next career move to wondering whether I was going to survive this current episode. I now faced a three-week wait to find out if the dermatologist had been successful in completely taking out the cancerous area, and to be sure it hadn't spread to my lymph nodes.

I was due back at work within the hour, but my job didn't matter to me: the only thing on my mind was to reach out to the people I loved. I hadn't told friends or family that I was waiting for the outcome of a biopsy. I didn't want to worry anyone. I had also assured myself that it would be fine. Now I had the results, and it felt like a burden I needed to share.

I pulled my phone from my pocket and instinctively called the one person I knew who only ever played to win. My dad had never been someone who was entirely comfortable with talking on an emotional level, but just then I needed his fighting spirit. He was shocked when

I blurted it all out, at a loss as to what to say, unlike my mum when I spoke to her. She spoke positively about the fact that it had been caught now, and that we would face this together. It was good to talk to both of them. I was frightened, and was looking at a time of huge uncertainty, but was comforted to know that I didn't have to confront it alone.

I've always considered myself as having a positive outlook. Following my diagnosis, however, I couldn't help but fear the worst. Despite my doctor's assurance that we just needed to wait and see, I found it very hard to stop dwelling on the worst-case scenario. I'd also been advised that I might be required to undergo further treatment. Frankly, that terrified me. I felt powerless and paralysed by uncertainty.

Just to make that time even more challenging, following the removal of the melanoma, the dermatologist had instructed me to avoid strenuous activity for three weeks. I had stitches from the operation and the wound needed to heal. That meant no more coaching, personal training or even working out on my own. Even though it was only a small (and, hopefully, temporary) change to my lifestyle in the big scheme of things, it came as a huge blow. I also didn't feel comfortable telling everyone at the gym the reason why I had to clear my timetable for that period. Somehow, I thought people might think of me as 'ill' and change the way they related to me. It had come as such a surprise that I wasn't ready to deal with it publicly. In that time, I also pulled out of social events I had planned with friends. I pretty much went dark. I confided in my boss, who assured me I could have all the time off I needed, but as it didn't affect my office work, I just carried on as normal.

Everything had changed for me in a heartbeat, yet there I was at my desk as usual. I was pushing paperwork and making calls. Only now it seemed as if a filter had been removed from my vision. With an awareness that life was very precious, and that mine might well be on the line, my City work seemed completely meaningless to me. If I really did just have a couple of months or years to live, did I want to use that by making money out of money? At the time, I was in no position to act. Now was not the moment to make huge changes when I had an illness to fight. I kept telling myself that this nightmare could all be over by the time I next visited the dermatologist. So, I returned for the follow-up consultation with an open mind yet clung to the hope that I'd receive the all-clear. Instead, the results of my last biopsy revealed that the dermatologist would need to go deeper with a further procedure.

In the months that followed, my family and I played a kind of race and chase against the skin cancer. While my mum was there for me to talk things through, my dad came into his own as my rock. He attended every consultation with me, wrapped his arm around me when I needed it and basically treated this illness as something we could beat as a team. It brought out a side to him I hadn't seen before and helped us to connect on a deep level. I have so much respect for my parents, as well as my sisters, for everything they did for me throughout that time. When things go wrong, I was reminded that love is unconditional in families – whether it's the one we're born into or those that we create through shared values and passions.

In total, I went through three operations and additional plastic surgeries to deal with what was effectively a chunk removed from my lower back. Time effectively went on hold for me throughout this period. I went to work, rested, talked to my parents and those friends who knew, and promised myself that, if things worked out, I would never waste another day of my life. It was a big promise, but in moments of darkness it gave me a point of light to focus on. And I also owed a debt of gratitude for the kindness and honesty of the client at my class who stepped forward and saved my life. In all honesty, without her intervention I would have ignored the signs. If there's one thing I have taken away from that whole experience, it's a passion for encouraging anyone with concerns to check in with their GP. It doesn't take much, even if you need a second opinion to put your mind at rest. It could save your life.

Towards the end of my limbo period, in which I just felt like I was at the mercy of medical results, I received an invitation from Peloton to travel to New York for an audition. With all that was going on, I had all but forgotten about my meeting with Cody, as well as the film I'd recorded and submitted. So, when they responded after a long silence to ask if I would be interested in exploring a way forward, it came as a surprise. It wasn't until I checked in with the dermatologist for what would be a critical consultation that I saw it as some kind of sign that an end to this ordeal was in sight.

'Ben, you can relax,' he said. 'The latest biopsy came back. For the first time, we can be cautiously optimistic.'

It was news I just hadn't dared to dream about.

The cancer appeared to have gone, with no need for further treatment but rather close monitoring for some time to come. The dermatologist framed his prognosis with huge caveats. We needed to be vigilant, he said, and prepared for setbacks. Even so, he had given me enough hope to feel reborn, and I left the clinic to begin what felt like my second life. Having been inactive for so long, I was desperate to get back to the gym. It was in that space, I had come to realise, where I felt I truly belonged.

When I look back on that short, frightening period of my life, I see it now as a game changer. Before my diagnosis, I was leading two lives. One provided me with security and career prospects. The other rewarded me in more meaningful ways.

I just loved coaching and fitness, but I had been reluctant to make the leap completely into that world. It would mean giving up a decent salary and the stability that came with being on a solid rung on the career ladder. Quite simply, I was scared to make a change and upset the status quo. But now I'd been forced to consider the passing of time and how you spend it as something that was truly precious, and my serious health scare gave me the push I needed.

Having been given this chance, my eyes were wide open to what was important. If I only had three years to live, why would I want to spend it sitting at a desk? Every minute of each day was valuable, not something I wanted to waste again. At work in the office, I spent time investing in businesses rather than truly engaging with the people within them. That job had lost its appeal. I wasn't fired up by it. Whereas the prospect of a career in fitness made me feel alive. Essentially, everything was pointing me in the direction to make the transition, but only I could act on that.

When I talked to my dad about how my perspective on life had changed, I thought he would just encourage me to focus on my career in the City and let normality return. Before I was ill, I had told him about my growing interest in coaching. Back then, his view was that I needed to think long term and ask myself whether that kind of work was sustainable. This time, when I revealed that I'd been approached by a pioneering company that took fitness, technology and community to a new level, he told me to follow my heart.

'If it makes you happy,' he replied, in a conversation that meant so much to me, 'then go for it.'

Within a week, I was pretty clear in my mind that I was doing the right thing, when I found myself in a New York gym rigged with cameras and studio lighting, preparing to audition as a coach in front of the powers that be at Peloton.

I had chosen not to tell them about what I'd recently been through. I was still coming to terms with the fact that I might just have put the cancer behind me. As that came with no guarantees, it would take some time before I would be able to talk about it in the past tense. All I wanted to do was focus my attention on becoming as fit and healthy as possible, on my own terms, so that I could throw myself into this great opportunity. I had also really missed the simple act of movement. All too often we take for granted the fact that movement of any kind is a blessing, until it's taken away. Now that it was available to me once more, I was keen to share the benefits with others. Our health is both precious and enriching. For me, it had become the definition of wealth, and something that filled me with gratitude every day. With this renewed outlook, I wanted to make a difference to people's lives by bringing them together in a community built on shared values.

As the cameras rolled, I hoped that burning passion I felt would shine through.

*

THE GREAT ESCAPE

Often, when we're feeling down, bored or in need of distraction, we reach for our phones. We spend a little time online and with our social media, and that short escape from the real world provides a natural high.

Dopamine is a chemical substance released in the brain. It serves important functions throughout the body by sending messages through nerve cells, one of which is to influence our mood and help us to feel good. A dopamine hit can provide a lift, so we feel better about ourselves, but it's only temporary. It also doesn't resolve the reason why we picked up our phones in the first place. As a result, we keep on escaping from the world around us by spending time with our small screens.

In my view, that's not sustainable. Essentially, we need to revisit the concept of happiness, recognise its value and work to place it at the heart of our lives.

Today, we are never far from our phones. They play an important role, but the relationship we've formed with them is one small example of what I consider to be an instant gratification crisis. We might feel good for a moment as we check our posts for likes, but we also know that social media can spark all manner of anxieties and insecurities. Life can be hard and, unless we find constructive ways to make the most of it, the temptation arises at times to block it out.

During my first few years in finance, when I wasn't prepared to recognise that I was struggling to cope, I fell into a pattern of working and partying hard. I didn't use my free time to recover and recharge.

I simply went out because I hoped it would make me happy. Sure enough, I had a great time drinking and clubbing until the early hours, but with work in the mix it couldn't last. If anything, as my sleep, fitness and diet suffered, it made the problem worse. Stress can affect us in all sorts of ways and, over that period, it crept up on me both mentally and physically. I had focused all my energies in trying to promote myself as a success story, but frankly on the inside I was miserable.

We are better than this. We only have one life, after all. Good health and happiness – which we can consider as one – isn't a given, and I learned the hard way that neglecting it can only lead to one outcome. Ultimately, we owe it to ourselves to find the kind of contentment that's deep, sustainable and doesn't just benefit us but also the wider world. Financial wealth is just one part of this equation. No matter what our background, we all have the power to look at ways that we can be sure we're aligned with our values and actively seek long-term happiness over materialistic or short-term hits.

It's one thing to look up from our phones, but what are we seeking once we've opened our eyes to the world around? It's all too easy to set up unrealistic expectations of what true happiness means. The temptation to measure it in terms of money, property, career success or social-media popularity is hard to ignore, but essentially risks leaving us feeling insecure, frustrated and anxious. We have even found ourselves living at a time when our physical appearance has become a factor in determining our status. It's easy to think that a defined set of abs or glutes, a fake tan or bleached teeth – which are all effectively cosmetic interventions by another name – will somehow make us more desirable or worthy of attention. The fact is it's all just window dressing when, ultimately, what matters is the heart and soul inside us. It's my belief that true happiness comes from setting aside such expectations and focusing on the simple aspects of our lives that we may take for granted but, without which, we couldn't manage. For me, I'm talking about love, companionship, an active life and shared experiences that enrich my existence every single day.

It took a serious health scare for me to come to appreciate the meaning of true happiness, and that began with practical steps to optimise my health. I had no interest in bodybuilding to look good. Instead, I focused on building the body that would help me to make the most of my existence. Just then, any concept I had of looking good had to begin by feeling great. From shaping up my diet to cutting out factors that caused me stress, ring-fencing good sleep patterns and simply coming to appreciate the people and pursuits in my life that mattered to me, my life improved considerably.

OUTER JEWELS, INNER EMPTINESS

Throughout my career as a fitness coach, I have visited many gyms. They've come to signpost my journey in some ways. As a result, some are deeply significant to me. The boutique gym that hosted the first indoor cycling class I ever attended is a case in point. It was really just a basic space, yet both warm and inviting. It was there that I came to recognise the draw behind getting active in a group situation. It wasn't just the shared motivation but the friendships I formed with people from all walks of life. In the same way, I have fond memories of my time working out in the rundown little space on the ground floor of the Parisian apartment block. At the time, I was lost and quite lonely, and it was there that I first began to recognise that everything would be OK. The equipment wasn't up to much, but that place became somewhere I could work on both my body and mind.

In my experience, gyms such as this possessed heart. There was just something about them that drew me in and helped me to grow. The equipment was basic, but I brought the commitment to make the most of it. My goal was to build a healthy body and that was something money couldn't buy. It came down to time, passion and determination, which are qualities only we can bring to the game. Regardless of wealth, race or background, everyone comes into the gym on an even playing field. It falls to nobody else but us to work hard to build our minds and bodies to the best of our abilities.

The energy of a gym is built by the people within and I've seen the flipside in many hotel gyms around the world. Lots of them can dazzle with the latest kit under state-of-the-art mood lighting and with mirrors angled to make everyone look awesome. Yet without the regular faces and the shared commitment of going there frequently, they often lack soul. There's no community or sense of shared interest. These ventures will rarely inspire people to make long-term change because there's no sense of belonging or continuity.

It means people come and go, but there's no chatter or smiles. Nor is there a sense of community. Everyone just plugs into their ear buds, cutting themselves off from their surroundings, and then leaves, as swiftly as possible as it's been a chore and not a pleasure. I suspect for many it's a one-off visit, a place to escape the stress of a busy job, or a short burst to get fit, rather than something that becomes central to their routines. No matter how much money has been thrown at these projects, it's all surface – and that troubles me.

I also see it as a warning for those who live their lives at a surface level. Leasing a flash car might earn attention and project an image of success, but if we can barely afford it, what's the point? It just wouldn't make me happy. If anything, it would leave me feeling anxious.

Even in our consumer culture, I strongly believe it's still possible for us to see beyond it all and find true, meaningful and lasting happiness. If we can break away from the need for what I call the outer jewels and establish a sustainable form of wellbeing, the need for instant gratification just fades away. I'm not proposing a cure for all ills here. Just a reframing of how we live our life to place our values at its heart and instil purpose moving forwards.

A WAKE-UP CALL FOR US ALL

What does sustainable happiness mean? We can't guarantee that the sun will shine every day, after all. Some aspects of our life are completely out of our control. We've seen that setbacks and challenges can occur at any time and, though we can become equipped with strategies to overcome them, it's admittedly hard to stay smiling, having tumbled down the mountain for the umpteenth time. Smart thinking and a willingness to consider alternative approaches, along with grit and determination, take over at those times, of course. That means being prepared for all eventualities and, in some ways, this is key to the kind of happiness that can last a lifetime.

Let's take ageing as an example. When we're young, the prospect of playing with our grandchildren can seem so far away that it's not relevant to our current lives. The trouble is that, if we don't look after ourselves today, we could be storing up problems for the future. Our health, fitness and welfare are all key here. By placing them centre stage, we're not just able to live our best lives in the here and now – it also sets us up for the future. Personally, I want to be able to be active in my later life, and I can give myself every chance of achieving that. It's an investment, much like a pension, only it doesn't have to cost us a penny. What's more, it's never too late to start. Despite the challenges that come with shifting habits towards an active life, there will always be benefits ahead. So, start today.

Our health and fitness are also very easy to neglect, as I found out for myself at a time when work seemed to dominate my days. I just wasn't in the right frame of mind to think beyond instant gratification because, deep down, I was so unhappy.

Then I received a skin cancer diagnosis, and everything changed.

As wake-up calls go, it was a loud one.

When the doctor laid out the worst-case scenario, it forced me to look at my lifestyle in a different light. While he made it clear that cancer can strike for all sorts of reasons, I couldn't help but feel as if I was partly to blame. I'd spent years feeling massively stressed, and basically neglecting my health and welfare, and now here I was processing the fact that my lifespan could be limited. I vowed to change.

I can now see that I was seeking some kind of control at a time when I felt so helpless. I looked at my life and recognised aspects where I could take charge. I wanted to make positive changes where possible, and effectively optimise my health and wellness so I stood the best chance of beating this illness. From that moment on, I knew I would never take my health for granted again.

Despite the fact that I had found myself in a frightening situation, it actually came as a relief for me to put my fast living behind me. It took a cancer diagnosis for me to recognise that I wasn't enjoying it. I looked back on my habit of overworking and partying hard only to realise how miserable I had become. I had strong values. I'd grown up with a desire to be passionate about life, caring and committed, and had ended up neglecting friends and family in a bid to chase impossible work deadlines, then escape from it by clubbing. That wasn't the person I wanted to be, and now I had a compelling reason to reshape my act. As I got over the shock of my diagnosis, I set out to maximise my chances of beating it with a razor-sharp focus.

In rebuilding and refining my lifestyle, I had two goals. Above all, I was determined to beat cancer. I was in the care of a great dermatologist and my family were there for me throughout. Aware that it had taken an illness for us to come together, I wanted to be a team player, and that meant getting myself into the best shape in terms of my health and wellbeing. At the same time, it became clear to me that focusing on becoming the best version of myself could bring me the kind of inner happiness I had been lacking for so long. As I started to make improvements to everything from my diet to my fitness and sleep, I felt better in every way. I had a battle on my hands, but I didn't just want to be strong enough to beat cancer. I intended to keep living my life in this way because it put me in such a positive frame of mind, helped me to recognise what was truly rewarding and prepared me for every eventuality.

It took an illness for me to bring my life into focus and encourage me to draw my values to the fore. Without it, I might not have made the leap from finance to fitness. In doing so, it liberated me from chasing quick fixes in a bid to feel better about myself. Why? That change came as I found myself and, following the all-clear from my dermatologist, I have never looked back. My awakening was a response to an emergency situation, but it's one that each of us can undertake at any time. We're talking about a process here. It's available to everyone and requires just one condition: we have to recognise that happiness comes from within.

AUDITING OURSELVES

Each day presents us with a range of decisions to make. What we eat, how we spend our time, who we spend our time with. Stress is an inevitable part of life. Some stress can positively motivate us. However, when a stressful situation is going on, or we are experiencing multiple layers of stress, we need to equip ourselves with the best tools to manage it. Our ability to manage stress often comes down to if, and how, we are balancing the energy givers and energy takers in our lives.

Energy givers are things like healthy food, sunshine, fresh air, meditation, healthy relationships, hydration, music, reading, rest, movement and nature. Energy takers are things such as people-pleasing, too much screen time or social media, overthinking, junk food, no exercise, dehydration, overworking, sitting for too long, and so on. Our overall wellbeing is directly related to how well we manage the energy in our lives and being aware we should make changes when things aren't feeling right. It's a constant balancing act between pushing yourself to 'RAISE THE BAR' and make the most of life, and making sure you are recharging and filling up your cup as and when you need.

Struggling with my mental health while working in finance and being diagnosed with skin cancer prompted me to undergo a comprehensive review of my lifestyle. Over the last ten years, both working as a high performing employee within a private equity firm and as a Peloton instructor, I have been testing and trialling various wellbeing practises with the aim of improving my mood, energy levels and overall performance in life. I am not a doctor or an expert, so I can only tell you what has and hasn't worked for me and my clients, but I've outlined below some of the key focus points in 'Raising the Bar' for yourself. I by no means expect us to be perfecting these every day, but it's an amazing toolkit to tap into as you go through life. In auditing myself, I typically work on four general areas that have contributed to an overall improvement in my wellbeing: Movement, Food, Rest and Mental Wellbeing.

AUDITING YOUR WELLBEING

Movement

This is the non-negotiable one for me. Keeping up with your physical wellbeing can improve your immune system, reduce stress, boost your energy levels and help you feel more confident.

Physical activity has a direct impact on mental wellbeing, and vice versa. You don't have to be a natural exerciser to be active. I've seen clients start small and build up their confidence to be a regular 'exerciser' by gradually building healthy habits into their lifestyle. It's amazing to witness. Here are the things I focus on when I'm trying to regain control over my exercise regime:

1. **Staying active can be any form of exercise.** Make a commitment to move your body every day. From a walk to a Peloton class and anything in-between, it's important to choose exercise that you enjoy, mix things up and remember exercise is a mood boosting treat, not a punishment.

2. **Find a workout partner or community.** Finding a group of people who shared similar interests and goals to me transformed my perception of health and fitness. It's also an amazing way to keep on track on the days I don't feel like going and stay motivated to set personal goals for myself.

3. **Consistency is key in getting results.** Twenty minutes of walking is better than none. Results don't come overnight. It requires hard work and consistency to build a stronger you. Blocking time out of my diary for a workout and treating it as non-negotiable, like an important work meeting, can be a gamechanger in prioritising my health. I must admit, this is

the one I struggle with most, and therefore try to prioritise it even more.

4. **Having training-specific goals.** Think running a marathon, or lifting a specific weight when deadlifting. These goals can be, and should be, unique to you, depending on what it is you're wanting to achieve. Building a workout plan around these specific goals can result in better results. Moving away from aesthetic goals and focusing on building a body that can function well has been a gamechanger for me. I want to be active with my future kids and grandkids for as long as possible, so longevity is my driving force when picking training goals.

5. **You can't out-train a bad diet.** For me, feeling great is a combination of exercise and good food. In order to perform well, I need to nourish my body with food that is going to energise me. There isn't much sustainability in doing five workouts a day to try and hit a particular weight or fitness goal and then feeding your body crap. Mental clarity is what keeps me on track with my exercise regime and I believe that is from the food I am eating.

6. **Music and movement combined is medicine for the mind and body.** Having a playlist full of 'belters and bangers' to work

out to makes workouts more enjoyable. Moving your body should be fun. Music is an amazing motivator and makes the workout time fly by.

7. **Get kitted out.** There is something to be said about investing in good quality sportswear. It's not about the brand or price tag itself, but more about the way it makes you feel. The confidence builds when you're taking pride in how you're showing up in this area of your life. This is you identifying as someone who cares about being active.

8. **Reminding myself that 'self love is never selfish' when it comes to health and wellbeing.** We can't expect to show up for our loved ones around us if we aren't willing to prioritise building ourselves up first. Don't wait until it's too late to start looking after yourself. Take a moment for you.

Food

We could argue that our relationship to fast food is part of our instant gratification crisis. It's quick and easy, and provides a taste hit and energy boost when we're too busy (or lazy) to cook for ourselves. The downside is that a lot of fast food is high in sugar, refined oils, salt and saturated fat that can cause inflammation in our bodies. It can also be low in antioxidants and fibre, which makes it fine for the occasional treat, but far from optimal for our health if it becomes a regular feature in our diets.

Working long hours in my finance job, I felt like I didn't have enough time to cook. Eating became a chore to me, and the quickest way to tick it off the list was by ordering in, and snacking on multiple protein bars. As a result, my diet took a nosedive.

Yet again, it wasn't until I made the change that I came to realise what a profound effect a good diet can have. I created time to cook for myself, and even found that I enjoyed it. I wasn't just fuelling better, but also discovering a passion for something I had previously just overlooked. It became a challenge and an opportunity to shape up a diet that supported my new lifestyle, and I loved it.

Good nutrition means doing our best to eat a balanced diet. First things first, what works for me may not work for you, as all our bodies are a different, but as a nutrition coach and through my own experience with how food makes me feel, the following are some key areas that I like to focus on when 'Raising the Bar' in my nutrition:

1. **Load up on H$_2$O and electrolytes.** Drinking enough water through the day doesn't just help digestion, but also encourages clear thinking and helps to regulate mood swings. Ensuring I drink a minimum of two to three litres of water

a day is something that transformed my concentration while working in finance and has aided my performance as an athlete and Peloton instructor. We lose salts and minerals through sweating and an imbalance can leave us feeling rubbish. I always have electrolyte tablets on the go with me, adding them to my water when needed.

2. **Always read the labels.** A lot of the food we see in our supermarkets is packed with hidden refined sugar and vegetables oils that are causing inflammation in our bodies. The low-fat options of foods are often stripped of the goodness and a lot of low-calorie options are filled with chemicals that are messing with our gut health. I have moved away from focusing on calories and like to focus on limiting the chemicals that are in the food I eat. Being aware of what I was putting in my body transformed the way I shopped and by making simple and easy swaps for more foods in their original form, I was able to change my energy and mood levels for the better.

3. **Focus on adding foods, not eliminating them.** One of the things I've loved learning most is not to restrict myself, but instead to reduce the highly processed foods that can land on our plates too often. My focus is a plate of food that loves me back. Fill your plate with vegetables, grains, legumes, fruits,

nuts, meats, seafood, herbs, spices, garlic, and eggs. The more you add these foods to your plate, the less space there is for the bad stuff.

4. **Building your recipe library.** Collecting a good range of quick and easy healthy recipe ideas has given my partner and me inspiration to make sure we are eating a diet that's diverse and interesting. The internet and social media are two amazing places to discover new recipes.

5. **Gut-healthy foods that love you back.** Eating food as close to its natural state as possible has been a gamechanger for my mood and energy levels. Colourful vegetables and fruits are loaded with prebiotic fibre, vitamins, minerals, and antioxidants, many of which have potent health effects. You hear the term 'eat the rainbow' – it's true. Colour on the plate is key. Herbs and spices are not only amazing for adding flavour, but also add nutrient density to each meal. Your gut will love foods like yogurt, kefir, miso, sauerkraut, kimchi, almonds, olive oil, kombucha, garlic and ginger.

6. **Organic over non-organic.** Organic food may be a bit more expensive, but the produce you are eating has a higher nutrient content as the food is grown in better soil conditions. This option isn't always available for many

different reasons, but if you can, this is an investment your body will thank you for.

7. **Increase your protein intake.** Protein is needed for growth and repair of body tissues and is especially important for healthy muscles and bones. I always try my best to choose lean proteins: lean beef, Greek yogurt, fish, lentils/beans/ peas, chicken, pork, eggs, nut butters and prawns. If you want to build and maintain muscle mass, a focus on protein is important.

A healthy diet can be achieved with clear information and can also be done on a budget. Good nutrition benefits every aspect of our life so that we can crack on and make the most of it.

Rest

I used to believe it was something I could minimise in order to make the most of my working day. The way I saw it, sleep just took up time I needed to get on top of all the work mounting up on my desk. Yes, it might've created more waking hours, but looking back it gave me no advantage. Tired, irritable and emotional, I struggled to focus and found myself prone to moments of high anxiety. Practices that have benefited my rest regime are the following:

1. **Developing good sleep hygiene.** Quality is key here. For me, it's very simple. Sleep is key to a long and healthy life, and while it's easy to neglect, there are huge benefits from optimising that down time. Creating a consistent sleep routine, avoiding technology in (at least) the hour before bed, wearing blue light blocking glasses, creating a restful sleeping environment, taking time to wind down and avoiding stimulants, alcohol and/or spicy food prior to going to bed can help you get the quality of rest you deserve.

2. **Hot and Cold Therapy.** Going from a sauna into an ice bath. A hot shower into a cold shower. A hot bath on its own. There are various ways to get the benefits here, and there is not a one size fits all approach to this. When I use this practice regularly, this is something that transforms my mood and energy levels, improves circulation, relieves muscle soreness and improves mental clarity. If you haven't tried it, you are missing out.

3. **Breathwork.** I'm terrible at sitting still. I never understood or could get into meditation. However, breathwork for me is more of an active form of meditation. Deep breathing and relaxation activate the other part of your nervous system, the parasympathetic nervous system, which sends a signal to your brain to tell the anxious part that you're safe and don't need to use the fight, flight or freeze response. Deep breathing gets

more oxygen to the thinking brain. It's a tool I use to relieve anxiety or stress, but can be used anytime and anywhere.

Mental wellbeing

Our mental health is just as important as our physical health. This means that we should prioritise practices that boost our mental health and prepare ourselves with a toolbox of skills to help manage our stress containers. Self-care practices should be a priority in our everyday lives, and that doesn't just mean bubble baths and scented candles – though they can help. Self-care is a vital part of looking after your mental wellbeing, and some self-care strategies that have helped me boost my mental wellbeing have included:

1. **Be kind to yourself.** Focusing on calming stress hormones and regulating our nervous system means prioritising time and energy to activities that promote these things.

2. **Get tested.** Getting DNA and vitamin and mineral blood-tested allowed me to supplement knowing what my body needs, rather than taking what is marketed to me. Knowledge is power.

3. **Focus on good mood foods.** Make a mood food diary. List down how foods make you feel. Self-awareness is everything

when it comes to choosing foods that love you back and more awareness and information will allow you to make better choices, For me, getting rid of inflammatory foods in my diet was a gamechanger. Sugars and refined oils mostly. Adding gut-supporting foods has helped me regain my energy and focus.

4. **Getting connected with nature.** Getting sunlight in your eyes first thing in the morning is absolutely vital to mental and physical health. Even if it's two to ten minutes. It should be a non-negotiable for us all and has been a game changer for me. Having a dog and getting out for early morning walks has helped me with this hugely, but getting out into nature more often on the whole has had a dramatically positive impact on my mental and physical health.

5. **Fostering healthy, trusted social connections.** The correlation between strong social connections and happiness is clear. Whether it's a close friend, a family member or a registered therapist, having someone to air your thoughts and emotions to can be a game changer for managing anxiety and stress. Having friends and family to celebrate the small and big wins with in life is key. I've found it's important to be good to those that are good to you. In order to have good friends, colleagues and siblings, I need to show up as one. Don't shy away from

the hard conversations, and remember, nine times out of ten, the person on the other end of the phone will appreciate you opening up as they are having struggles themselves.

6. **Working towards a healthy work–life balance.** Schedule joyful and fun events with friends and family away from work. Celebrate the moments that deserve to be celebrated. Regardless of how big or small. Put the hard work in when you need to grind, but no job or salary is worth sacrificing the priceless moments in life.

7. **Learning when and who to say NO to.** I've spent time learning how my mind and body reacts to certain situations and how best to take accountability and actionable steps to protect my mental health. I've also started to find joy in missing out (JOMO). Don't subscribe to other people's definition of 'fun'. Fun doesn't have to mean partying, drinking or socialising. Fun can be doing a workout with friends, solitude, getting immersed in a book, or working on a passion project. Fun is yours to define.

These four areas combine to provide the foundation for great wellbeing. Without one, the others fall. So it's vital to implement strategies that boost each area, and not focus all our attention on just one. Making some of these gradual healthy changes in our day-to-day lives can quickly provide huge benefits in return.

ENDURING HAPPINESS

Let's be clear, happiness isn't something we can buy or manufacture. We can have all the trappings of success, from the career to the car, and yet feel empty inside. In the same way, we can't force ourselves to be happy – that has to come from within. What we can do is create the right environment in which it can grow.

Running an audit on our lives to date is an effective way to assess where we are in life. Are we truly happy, or is there work to be done? Whatever the case, a change for the better is always possible, and we should never lose sight of the fact that help and support is always out there if we need it. Whether it's someone we know or a trusted professional, opening up about what's going on in our hearts and minds is an effective way to bring the light in if we need it. Following my cancer treatment, and in making the move from finance to fitness, I hired a life coach to advise me. As well as seeking to understand myself and establish what had become a new normal in terms of my lifestyle, I sought advice on how to make such a big career change. My aim was to be as productive as possible, but also in control of work. It had come to dominate my life in the City and, if I stood any chance of lasting happiness, that had to change, which it did.

In the end, we're seeking the kind of enduring contentment that comes from knowing that we strive to be our best selves. We may not feel on top form all the time, of course. What matters is that we build a life rich in meaning, love and purpose, so that every experience has value – now and in the future.

RAISE THE BAR: MILESTONES

- We need to revisit the concept of happiness and prioritise meaningful and sustainable contentment over instant gratification.
- Good health and happiness are indivisible.
- Reviewing our lifestyles on a regular basis, and making adjustments and changes as we develop, allows us to be the best version of ourselves. Ultimately, this is key to lasting inner happiness.
- Auditing our wellbeing doesn't mean ticking off every wellbeing practice available to us every day of our lives, but instead having awareness of the tools available to us and making a conscious effort to tap into them as regularly as we can to raise the bar for ourselves.

PART 4

RAISING THE BAR

*I have learned that passion counts for everything
as we find out feet, along with a willingness to learn – not
just from knowledge but setbacks and mistakes.*

CHAPTER 9

BECOMING YOUR BEST SELF

In order to be the best version of ourselves,
we need to start from a place of honesty.

I was a pioneer. That was how it felt to me when I auditioned to become a coach with Peloton. The concept of hosting classes online and interactively, in a way that connected people all around the globe, was completely new. In New York, the team I met were faced with tackling obstacles and devising solutions that just hadn't existed until this time, which made it hugely exciting.

In this unknown territory, in which an open mind and willingness to collaborate was key, only one thing was certain to me: in order to make it a success, everyone had to give 100 per cent of their energies. In my case, that meant learning to work with a camera. It was something I'd never done before, but I was determined to master it. With the help of an excellent crew, I absorbed their advice and guidance in order to project myself in a way that was both confident and approachable. We all knew it wasn't a polished performance because effectively it would be the start of a learning process. It meant I needed to be humble enough to recognise when I sucked, and determined to improve, while knowing at all times that I had all the tools and support that I needed to make that happen. Had I come in hoping to be the consummate showman, it just wouldn't have worked. We were all new to the game. What mattered is that we were able to learn together and play as a team.

Away from the audition, I spent a few days meeting other key members of the company. We effectively assessed each other, and I flew home hoping that we had forged a connection. With first-hand experience of how it worked in America, I couldn't help feeling that my late grandfather would have been fascinated. He had been quite an early adopter of technology. He embraced email when most older folk were still dubious. I felt sure he would have loved what Peloton represented, not least because it placed community at its heart.

Having flown out to New York with an open mind, I returned to the UK with high hopes. I really wanted to be part of the journey that Peloton were about to embark upon. I had to fly back to the States one more time for a meeting that felt like a make-or-break assessment and had to struggle to keep it together when they offered me the job. When I called my dad, I found it hard to describe my role. It was one of those positions that would develop over time and I was fully invested in that ride.

I didn't enjoy handing in my notice back at the finance firm in London. My boss had given me a break at a challenging time in my career. I hoped that I had repaid him with hard work, but my departure wasn't part of his long-term plan. At the same time, he knew exactly what I'd been through and so, when I told him that I needed a change of direction, he understood. I was so grateful to him for everything he had done and, having worked through my notice, I left on good terms. I did wonder if he thought I would soon be knocking at his door again: I was walking away from a well-paid career in finance to become a coach for a fancy fitness company which hadn't even launched in the UK. I could understand why such a move might take people by surprise. It appeared to be such a massive leap of faith and yet, having lived with cancer, I knew what power that possessed. So, I returned to America to begin my training with not one cloud of doubt in my mind. This was the right thing for me at this time, no matter what the future had in store.

Within a very short time after landing in the States, and having settled into an apartment kindly provided by Peloton, I was back at the studio. It was great to see Cody again, who was central to the programme, and I didn't want to let him down. There was just so much to do in terms of training, with 12 weeks of intensive learning ahead of me, and I welcomed it. While I was fascinated by the whole induction into this new world, above all it meant I had no time to dwell on what had been a traumatic experience. I wanted to be busy, and not staring at a wall reflecting on a frightening illness, so I threw myself into the process.

As well as getting into really good shape, I had to learn how to host classes that would be live-streamed around the world. That meant learning to work with the camera as well as finding my voice with the help of a coach. The producers would record each significant run-through, and then we'd sit down to analyse it. We'd look at strengths and weaknesses at a detailed level and aim to make every step a learning experience. It was a deeply rewarding journey, and one that also helped me to understand myself further.

Peloton sets out to offer a stable of trainers comprised of distinctive personalities. The aim is to provide a broad choice appealing to a wide audience. It's also a fine art, as I discovered when it came to finding my place on the team. So, as part of my training, I embarked on a deep dive into what made me tick.

Peloton does a great job of encouraging us to figure out who we are and what we represent on the platform. They want us to be ourselves, to be authentic. That's really important to them – as much as it is to me. As a result, we talked about my background and experiences along with my outlook on life and the values that had guided me. It was useful to Peloton in terms of pitching me as: *'the British athlete and finance star from England set to jump into a workout with you'*. In summing up my journey in a snappy sentence, it also helped me to feel confident that I had something distinctive to offer. What I didn't throw into this mix, however, was the fact that I was in remission from skin cancer. Even though I would finally go on to embrace it as a critical part of my story, it still felt too raw. For all the hours I was putting into training, in the back of my mind I was quietly processing what I'd been through. Everyone is different in how they deal with life-changing events like serious illness. Personally, I didn't want to make it my top priority. I needed other goals to focus on while I made sense of it in the background.

In that three-month training period, I was acquiring a raft of new skills. For someone who had set out to make a career in finance, it was a whole new world. Despite my love of coaching, I found the performance aspect to be challenging. Working with multiple cameras, I had to learn when to switch my attention from one lens to the other without missing a beat – and all the while doing something intensely physical.

As much as I loved the work, I also knew that I had a long way to go before I reached the highest standard. How did I know this? Because Peloton had recruited another British coach for the UK launch, and she was a natural.

Leanne Hainsby had trained with the Royal Ballet and worked as a stage dancer with artists such as Katy Perry and Taylor Swift. She'd spent much of her professional life performing, and simply dazzled the camera. The first time I watched her running through a coaching session at the studio, I knew I had my work cut out if I wanted to meet her standard. I was reminded of how I felt when I first started working in finance on the graduate scheme. I had a lot to learn and yet, this time, I could confide in my fellow trainee because she was lovely. Not only that, she was really supportive.

Leanne helped me to feel more comfortable as a performer, and I came to value her opinion. We were also two Brits far from home, on the same exciting journey into somewhat unknown waters. We shared similar values and the same passion for fitness. Over time, we grew closer as our training progressed towards live coaching sessions on the Peloton platform to an American audience. We looked out for each other and, when our working friendship evolved into a relationship, it felt like the most natural thing in the world. Leanne helped me to be myself, and still does to this day. I wouldn't be half the man and instructor I am today without her.

My first Peloton class took me back to all the stages in my life when I felt like I had to step up. From training with various sports teams to public speaking or hosting club nights, every situation was different and yet, each time, I had faced a bar that had been raised beyond my comfort zone. I may have been new to live-streaming a fitness session, but, I reminded myself, I was certainly experienced in putting myself in this vulnerable position. This time, with the training behind me, I just needed to have faith in myself. Above all, I really wanted to make a success of it.

I had come a long way to be here, physically and mentally. I had also learned a great deal along the way, and that included the fact that a passion for any pursuit was the only way to factor happiness into success. I truly believed in what I was doing, and used this as the foundation as I found my feet. The team at Peloton had done a great job in getting me up to speed as a coach on the platform, but that didn't stop me from striving to improve. After the first couple of sessions, for example, I reviewed the footage with my producer and recognised that I was leaning towards the kind of big delivery that my American colleagues did naturally. Partly this was down to the fact that I was training in the States and was immersed in that culture, but I also admired trainers like Cody. When we start out on any pursuit, it's often tempting to feel we need to be like those who have found success in that field.

As I realised quickly enough, while cringing at the review footage, there is a difference between being inspired by someone and copying them. I admired Cody's charm and confidence, but what I needed to do was find those qualities in myself. If I tried to be someone else, even just a little bit, I wasn't being genuine and that became my ultimate goal. It meant finding the confidence to try things in front of the camera and learn from the failures and successes. We just kept pushing, reviewing and refining until I found my true self. That came once I realised that being calm and assured had as much impact as being bold and vocal. As that was more in tune with my personality (and very British!), it helped me to relax under the studio lights.

Finding myself for the camera was a vital lesson for me. In order to be the best version of ourselves, we need to start from a place of honesty. This level of self-scrutiny is what led me to take on a life coach. I realised I needed help in transitioning from finance to fitness, simply because I was committed to maximising the potential of this opportunity.

Until that moment, my life in the City had been incredibly structured. I had to be at my desk at a particular time, where I checked in with a PA who controlled my appointments through the day. Peloton rolled in a way that depended upon me managing my own time. This was liberating in so many ways, but I was keenly aware that I lacked experience in how to make it work to the best effect. My life coach helped me to identify areas for improvement and also build on my strengths, which was just what I needed. It helped me to optimise my time, and with that came a sense of confidence that I was hitting all the right marks.

Twelve weeks after joining the Peloton family, during which I learned essential skills by coaching classes on the American platform, Leanne and I returned home for the UK launch. We both agreed that the experience had taught us more about ourselves than any other up to that point. We were also really excited by the prospect of coaching with a British audience.

While the company had found a footing in America, we were effectively ambassadors for the brand in this new territory, which brought a great deal of responsibility with it. As community was so important to Peloton, people were encouraged to talk to each other and provide feedback. I found that really useful in terms of meeting audience needs, but as the platform grew in popularity, it also introduced me to the fact that I was now leading a life in public. That meant my words and actions could be scrutinised. At first, I found that quite intimidating, as if it existed to trip me up. As I grew more comfortable in the role, however, I came to realise that as I strive to be kind and positive in how I live my life, ultimately, I had nothing to hide. This was a very different existence from the one I had left behind in the City and, while it took some time for me to make the transition from finance to fitness, I was finally able to spread my wings.

Back in London, towards the end of 2018, we pretty much had to start from scratch in launching Peloton in the UK. Ahead of the opening, Peloton had assembled a new team. It was modest in size and, while everyone was at the top of their game, our roles effectively demanded that we pulled together whenever we could to deliver on our shared vision. As the company was in the process of building a custom studio to live-stream classes, we found ourselves preparing to host the first sessions from a sound studio in East London.

The studio had lots of character as a location. It was just never designed to be a state-of-the-art fitness studio, and so we had to improvise. Leanne and I used caravans as changing rooms and had to learn not to touch the studio walls during a workout because it made them wobble. In those early days, when Peloton had only just made their bikes available in the UK, our audiences were relatively small. In some ways, that only encouraged me to put as much effort and enthusiasm into it as I could. The way I saw things, it was the surest way for word to spread that we had something special going on. It felt like we were growing a family, and everyone was welcome to come along for the ride.

During this time, Leanne and I were invited back to the States for a 'homecoming' event. Peloton invited over 3,000 members to New York to take part in classes and meet the instructors, giving everyone the chance to connect as a community. We assumed nobody would recognise us. We figured we'd stand in the background as the US instructors attracted all the attention, only to find queues of people wanting to meet us.

We were both blown away at the realisation that people were actually taking our classes from all over the world and had travelled in to say thanks and let us know how much they were enjoying what we were putting out there. It shone a light on the true power of this community and the unique nature of the individuals within it. We were really on to something, I realised, and we were only just getting started.

Seven months after we began in the UK, we swapped our fragile little home in East London for a studio in central London. For Leanne and me, it wasn't just the sudden upswing in building quality that came as a relief, but the travel, as our respective daily commutes were leading to long days. What's more, in a role that didn't have a template, we were discovering that the physical demands were having an impact on our bodies. Leanne and I were both young and fit, but recording so many workouts meant we were testing the same muscle groups. In particular, cycling is a great way to work on cardio, core and lower body strength. As a result, as well as finding time for rest and recovery and checking in with the physio to keep on top of things, we also had to make time in the gym to focus on upper body strength. So the move led to a reduction in commuting time and it improved our quality of life.

The new studio was in fact a halfway house. Peloton were still building what would become our permanent home in Covent Garden, and so our new studio was only ever temporary. It had sturdier walls and more space, which meant we could invite users to our classes. It reminded me of the old days, when I first fell in love with coaching, only now I was performing to a growing audience from all around the world. Leanne and I really felt like we had found ourselves as instructors and coaches, while Peloton's online community was helping to forge strong, supportive bonds between users. I remember once going into the studio and realising that it no longer seemed like a job. I loved being a Peloton coach and couldn't wait to see what would happen next. Our journey had only just begun and the global community was growing exponentially every day.

A few months into the new year, however, an international event, the repercussions of which no one could have anticipated, forced us to put our classes – and our lives – on hold. The pandemic. Covid-19. The world shut down.

The UK lockdown threatened to stop the wheels from spinning. Every single one of us had to make changes to our way of life in order to protect others and stay safe from the coronavirus. It was a testing time.

For businesses, many were presented with a choice between shutting down or adapting to a new way of life. And Peloton faced the challenge head on. We were all aware that we were living through a time when mental and physical health had never been more critical and believed that we could make a difference. As Leanne and I lived together and wanted to contribute, we offered to transfer our live-streamed classes from the gym to a back room in our flat.

On paper, it was simple. In reality, we had to learn a raft of new skills. We would have to become the technical team and somehow oversee filming, while hosting a class at the same time. With no guarantee that it would work, we persuaded the team to at least let us try. It had to be worth a shot; not just for us, but for the users at home looking to re-establish some structure to their lives. I don't think we anticipated what we'd let ourselves in for until we found ourselves picking through the boxes of camera and lighting equipment that arrived in our hall. Once we had set it up, our team were able to operate the equipment remotely, but we also had to troubleshoot any technical issues.

Our two-bedroom flat was a squeeze even before it doubled as a live-stream studio. We had a box room, which was used for storage, and so we cleared that out to create some space. It wasn't much. In fact, once the Peloton bike was in place there was barely enough room for the camera to get it all in frame. We operated from a laptop in the corner, which was just out of shot, and spent a while teaching ourselves how to light the space so it didn't cause huge shadows. It proved to be such a challenge, but with technicians on hand by phone and video call, we managed to pull something together that allowed us to keep the pedals turning.

Leanne and I hadn't been living together for long. Now we had to juggle roles, professionally and emotionally, in order to support each other. It meant I took care of the feed when she coached her session, and she did the same for me. In such a restricted space, I had to lie on the carpet with the laptop when Leanne was on camera in order to stay out of shot. When it was my turn in the saddle, I couldn't stand up without my head leaving the frame. Throw into that mix that we'd not made our relationship public to Peloton members yet so were double agents in that sense and you can see that we faced a string of hurdles, but as both of us believed that we could make it work, we just tackled them one by one.

We had to make sure our internet connection was robust enough to carry the live stream. Then we needed to learn how to coach wearing earbuds for the playlist, rather than playing it through loudspeakers, so we didn't disturb the neighbours. Sometimes one of us would have to sneak in to correct a mic, or the music would cut out and we'd be forced to improvise.

At times, it felt really frustrating. Just as we'd settled into spacious studios, here we were in a box room pretending to be professional. It was hard to tell how things were going. Our live streams were managed remotely, and so feedback was limited. I worried that our audience might be dwindling, but I was just thankful to be working. I only had to remind myself how lucky I was to double down on my commitment to making sure we were doing our very best under difficult circumstances.

While I was at home fretting that our sessions might appear shambolic, it seemed our users viewed them through a different lens.

Yes, things fell apart quite regularly, but Leanne and I were doing our best. Our enthusiasm never wavered, and I suppose that added a certain charm to the package. As a result, after months of live streaming from our box room, I was amazed to discover that we'd gone from hosting a few thousand global on-demand users per class to audiences of 100,000 upwards.

The numbers were mind-blowing. Without doubt, during lockdown the Peloton platform provided the perfect means for people to take part in exercise classes from home. As a result, demand for the bike rose massively, and I hope we played our part in connecting with those users and building the community.

Leanne and I both developed as coaches during this period. Lockdown forced us to be self-sufficient, to solve problems on our own and be innovative in our approach. Without professional lighting engineers, camera operators and the comfort of a producer to offer pointers, we had to take ownership of what we were doing. As we became aware of just how fast the community was growing, it felt like we were evolving from fitness coaches to leaders. People contacted us for training advice because they had nobody else to turn to and we rose to that challenge. Despite the compromises we had to make in live-streaming from home, the community really appreciated the fact that we had been prepared to just give it a go.

By the time the world began to open up, and we returned to the studio, I even felt a tinge of sadness. That time didn't just throw Leanne and I together. The Peloton community came with us on the journey. We had good times and testing moments throughout those months of isolation, along with a lot of laughs and good humour on all sides when live streams didn't quite go to plan. Above all, however, our coaching timetable provided structure for our members throughout that time, along with the connectivity to remind us all of something quite simple but true: together we are stronger.

*

ON HEART AND SOUL

As a schoolboy footballer, I would define success in one simple way. Through my young eyes, it was all about winning. That was it. Pure and simple. If my team came away victorious, I was happy, but what would really define it for me was if I had scored the winning goal. To find myself on the losing side was just unthinkable. I'd come off the pitch feeling like the last 90 minutes had been a complete waste of time.

It was only with age and experience that I came to appreciate that it wasn't the score that mattered, but the fact that I had put my heart and soul into the game. I was playing a sport that I loved and the reward was in knowing that I had shown commitment, teamwork and passion. This outlook didn't just apply to football, I realised, but to all aspects of life. Put simply, if I strive to be the best version of myself in everything I do, that sense of accomplishment is hard to beat.

At the same time, there is a great deal that we can do to shape and create a life that is both challenging and rewarding in equal measure. It all comes down to raising the bar, not just in terms of our life choices, but in what defines us as individuals.

INTENTION TO ACTION

I first experienced it in my year abroad at university, and then again when the shine came off my finance career. I'm talking about that nagging feeling that things could be better. It's something we're all familiar with. It can feel like we've travelled down the wrong path. Instead of being motivated to take on challenges to help us grow, it can seem like we're treading water just to stay afloat.

All too often, we do nothing about it. Instead of taking responsibility for the situation and making changes to our lives to allow us to thrive, we just press on with a sense of resignation. Frankly, we owe it to ourselves to be better than that.

We're not just talking about big life changes here. Often, we can have a clear sense of our values and yet fail to embody them. We all want to live in a world united by respect and consideration for each other, but how many times do we walk by litter on the street, dismissing it as somebody else's problem?

Making a change to little things like this can make as much of an impact as the larger transformations. Focus on what small steps you can make each day going forward. The compound impact of those actions can be seismic in a world in which good energy is contagious. In every case, however, that has to go further than just good intentions. It's easy to wish we had taken another career path or kid ourselves that we would pick up that discarded crisp packet if we weren't so busy. Intention is certainly key to becoming the best version of ourselves, but that can only be delivered by *action*.

So, let's look at how we can make it happen. Even though some changes for the better might be very simple, the fact that we don't often make them happen speaks volumes. In this view, let's begin by establishing strategies that take us all the way.

TURNING INTENTION INTO ACTION

Recognise the reward

Whether we're making minor tweaks to our behaviour in order to be true to our values or considering big changes, it's vital that we recognise our goal. This will become the source of our motivation and commitment, after all.

When it comes to small improvements in the way we live our lives, we often find reward both externally and internally. Let's say that I set out to make more time for the people I see regularly, but generally take for granted. It could be a neighbour who I pass on the street every day. Rather than walk on by, I smile and wish them a good day. It's a tiny adjustment, but one that invites a smile and cheery response, which makes us both feel good. As a positive affirmation it has long-lasting value. Why? Because it can only encourage me to build on a gesture that reflects my belief in spreading positive energy.

We're talking about tiny changes here, but collectively they can make a world of difference. I'm always mindful that, when I was diagnosed with cancer, people showed me nothing but kindness. It was something I came to really appreciate. I also wanted to follow that example and adopted the same outlook as I recovered. Today, working on a fitness platform with a global reach, I receive a steady stream of messages from people going through struggles in their lives who find solace and empowerment in my classes. It's humbling, and validates what I do, but I also strive to reply where possible, because kindness costs nothing and I know from experience that it can make a difference. Ultimately, it's these small, successive changes to our habits that can bring out the best in us all.

Bigger transformations demand more consideration from us. Like turning around a super tanker, it could take time and we have to plan in advance to cover every eventuality. We might also have to give up things in order to make a positive change to our lives, so it's important that it feels like the right move to make.

When Peloton approached me to join the team, I knew that fitness was a space that helped me to feel alive and happy. This was compounded by the fact that I'd spent several years in finance and was just coming through a serious illness that had forced me to ask myself what I really wanted to do with my life. Even so, I was daunted by the thought of moving from the City to the coaching class on a full-time basis. Even though I'd qualified to teach on a casual basis, this was a big leap.

It would have been easy to turn down the offer. Even though I didn't feel fulfilled by my finance job, it provided me with both security and familiarity. And yet I reminded myself that there was one asset missing from my life working as a private equity investor – happiness.

When evaluating whether to turn intention into action, we have to ask ourselves questions that are central to our lives. What do we want from the opportunity we face? What does it offer that will incentivise us to make it happen? All of us have different needs, of course. When it comes to career choices, for example, some of us prioritise money over everything else, and that is fine. Our appetite for risk is tied in here, and we need to be clear what we're prepared to take on.

In my case, I was prepared to forgo the City lifestyle and stability for the opportunity to build a career in a sphere I loved. For me, happiness was my priority. Yes, there was an element of risk involved, because at the time an interactive fitness platform was a pioneering concept, but having identified what it could bring me I felt it was one worth taking.

Recognising the reward is an effective motivator when it comes to turning our intent into action. At the same time, gathering as much insight and knowledge as we can allows us to make informed decisions that keep risk to a minimum. As a fallback plan, I had figured I could find another job in finance if things didn't work out. It wasn't something I would have relished doing. It just served as a safety net, which is another factor for consideration when it comes to making big life changes.

Don't burn bridges; build them

In order to become the best version of ourselves, often we need to let go of things that can leave us feeling anxious. From a steady income in changing careers to a relocation requirement away from friends and family, we're talking about things we might take for granted but which quietly provide us with certainty.

Often, the thought of losing these things can hold us back. Even if there are wider issues that are preventing us from embracing life, like a job we've outgrown, it's only natural that we think twice before walking away from a comfortable, if unfulfilling, environment.

In this situation, the smart move is for us to stop thinking about burning our bridges and focus instead on building them. When I moved to Peloton, I did so with some confidence that I could find my way back into finance if I needed to. Of course, I hoped it would be a one-way trip for all the right reasons. I also knew that I had picked up valuable interpersonal skills in my former industry that would carry forward in anything I chose to pursue. In terms of mindset, it allowed me to commit to the fitness industry without the anxiety of what I might do if it didn't work out.

Of course, it's not always possible or desirable to return to our former lives. If this makes the move feel too uncomfortable, consider ways to soften the landing. By the time Peloton invited me to join the platform, I had been coaching at a boutique gym on a casual basis for a couple of years. That gave me some insight into what the new role would be like. I also used the opportunity to grill my full-time colleagues about how such a role played out in reality. I wanted to know the pitfalls as much as the advantages, and in turn that clear picture of my landing zone made the jump less intimidating.

Sometimes there are ways to make big changes on a gradual basis, which allows us time to find our feet. If money is a concern, for example in starting up a new business, it's always worth considering supplementary work or a profitable side hustle as a means of supporting the venture. Whether it's financial peace of mind or a fact-finding mission to address any concerns, we can be creative in finding ways to build those bridges to the life we want to lead.

It's also worth stressing that often there is no rush to make a big change. In my finance role, we would take months looking into all aspects of a potential deal before making a commitment. We would want to be clear about every last deal and confident in what we were signing up to. Sometimes, after all the research, we would decide it wasn't the right fit. That didn't mean we had wasted our time. If anything, we had learned a lot from the process and become wiser for the experience. In other cases, of course, our efforts would lead to a deal that everyone could get behind because we knew it was the right thing to do. Ultimately, if we remind ourselves of our motivation for wanting to become the best version of ourselves, we will always find a way to make it happen. It all comes down to thinking smart about everything we do. There is huge joy to be had in being carefree and going with the flow, but there are also huge benefits in being diligent and feeling confident in our decisions and life choices. If we have done everything we can to make key decisions, we can feel confident that we made the right call at the time.

A better way of life

It takes courage to make changes to any journey or quest. Having set off on one path, and discovered it's not right for us, we find ourselves considering a new course that could bring upheaval to all aspects of life.

We know that establishing our motivation is as important as seeking smart ways to make the change in order to minimise risk and uncertainty. But the process doesn't end having made the leap. On the other side, we need to check in with ourselves on a regular basis to be sure we're making progress as expected. If we're hoping the opportunity allows us to grow and find true happiness, for example, that's something only we can interpret as individuals, or in conversation with a trusted friend or colleague. It requires pause for thought and absolute honesty, plus a willingness to keep on making small adjustments to stay focused on the end goal.

Life is a work in progress, after all. As our story evolves, so it can be that our values, aims and motivation develop. The best lives are those in which we are constantly challenged to grow, and sometimes that means we need to make further developments to support them. That's why it's so important to review how things are going on a regular basis and keep building on the experiences picked up on our journeys to inform the way ahead.

In raising the bar, we're making changes to our lives that allow us to fulfil our potential. Often, this can mean committing to a pursuit that started out as a personal passion. I fell in love with the gym long before I decided to place that at the heart of my profession, just as many people in creative industries like painting, photography or writing find a way to turn their interest into a fulfilling career. As a personal trainer, working in a space that is so important to me, I am excited about my next coaching session. I put my heart and soul into everything, from the playlist to the workout I have planned, because I want people to share my passion for fitness and health in a community environment. In my previous career, I grew to dread Monday mornings. In making a change for the better, I have never looked back.

Then there's music, which is key to the mix in which I work. I've always loved big tunes and live events that bring people together, ever since my student days at Leeds. At the time, I had no way of knowing it would become central to my fitness career, but it's allowed me to embrace a long-standing passion in a new and exciting way.

It's only right to flag up that, when we turn a personal project into a career or become dependent upon it for an income, that changes our relationship with it. At the end of a long day in finance, I used to race to the gym because that's how I unwound. Today, having pushed myself to deliver the best online workouts that I can, my out-of-work priorities have changed. Rather than stay at the gym, which is my equivalent of remaining at the office, I devote that time to friends and family. I do still like to work on my fitness outside of classes, but I'm mindful that my job is to keep my body in the right shape to keep delivering those workouts that so many people rely upon. As a result, I steer clear of contact sports like football and rugby simply because they carry a high risk of injury. I could see it as a sacrifice or rather remind myself that it allows me to build a career that brings me nothing but opportunities for growth, happiness and fulfilment.

RAISE THE BAR: MILESTONES

- Success can mean so much more than a financial return or trophies on the mantlepiece. Commitment, teamwork and passion can bring lasting rewards when it comes to any undertaking.
- When it comes to raising the bar, a series of small, considered or strategic steps can take us higher than just going for it and hoping for the best.
- Being true to our values is an effective goal in any situation, especially when facing challenges that allow us to live up to our true potential.

CHAPTER 10

PRACTISING GRATITUDE

Showing gratitude is our way of recognising
the value of happiness, which is what life is all about.

Peloton's purpose-built studios were a long time in the making, but it was worth the wait. When Covid closed down our makeshift home in London's Oxford Circus, our community of users was two million strong. By the time we began live streaming from our new UK HQ in Covent Garden, that figure had grown to five million.

It was a huge number, and with it came the responsibility to deliver. I wasn't daunted, however, because since Peloton came into my life, I have committed to giving 100 per cent to every session. I know how blessed I am to be in this position, and never take a moment for granted. It's like being at the pinnacle of a sport. There's no scope for simply showing up, and I love the commitment it demands. Knowing I've put everything I can into a class is just so rewarding.

As the world started turning once again, more instructors joined the platform. Peloton also strives for diversity, which is great to see, and that's given me the opportunity to learn from people from all backgrounds, cultures and walks of life. It's been lovely to see our family grow and embrace disciplines such as boxing, strength, yoga and running. As one of the longest-serving members of the UK team, which has grown from seven people when we launched to an 800-strong workforce, I also have responsibilities in training new coaches. Helping to bring out the best in them is such an honour and a pleasure for me. In doing so, I've come to realise that, in order to be a motivating force, we have to truly believe in our values. Not just those shared by everyone on the platform, but also on a personal level. If I look back on my formative years, I see a young man who pursued a childhood dream, discovered it wasn't for him and then overcame obstacles of every kind to find his true calling. My story taught me about resilience and determination, the strength that comes from loved ones and the fact that it's never too late to change direction in life to follow your heart.

Without any doubt, discovering I had skin cancer proved to be the wake-up call that ultimately changed my life for the better. It was a frightening experience, but opened my eyes to the fact that our time is precious. I had tried to get on top of a demanding job I didn't love, and that had led to burnout. Then I'd moved sideways. It offered the path of least resistance, but it was only my diagnosis that forced me to confront the fact that it wasn't my true calling.

The path to becoming a trainer wasn't easy. If anything, I could have stayed in my finance job, enjoying the salary and the trappings, but without any sense of true reward. Having made the leap, I will never forget what I left behind. It means I never take a day for granted, while staying grateful for the opportunity I have to live a fulfilling life.

Whatever is going on in my day, I have to be positive on the platform. I couldn't deliver unless it comes from the heart. It's my responsibility to the community, after all. They come to a class expecting me to bring energy and spirit as much as a workout. Of course, we all have stresses and strains that can cast a cloud over our day, but what matters is that I process these kinds of challenges in my own time. To help me get into the right frame of mind, I've come to rely on mantras. It could be a word or a phrase that I repeat to myself as a meditation. They tend to be positive in outlook, reminding me that I can face whatever task or challenge lies ahead with grace, courage and empathy for others. Often, I focus on a phrase that reinforces my efforts to put Peloton's members first in everything I do. It also comes from the heart. My mantras have to resonate with me. It's as if they're coded into my DNA, and I activate them by putting them into words. They're a like a gentle reminder to peel away any personal preoccupations or anxieties before we go live and just remind myself that I'm a good person underneath who wants to bring out the best in others. Recently, I was talking to someone who regularly attends my live-streamed class. She seemed surprised that I was approachable and friendly.

'You're as nice as you are on camera,' she said.

'Well, hopefully, because that's who I am,' I replied.

Frankly, I don't think I could pretend to be anyone else. It would be too exhausting and, to be honest, I like just being myself. I'm an instructor, not an actor. I had once tried to be a financial player, only to discover that it wasn't really me.

In striving to keep a positive mental attitude, I discovered the importance of being self-organised. Before I made the leap from finance to fitness coaching, my life was dictated by deadlines and client meetings. Most of these would be imposed upon me. I'd arrive at my desk to find my schedule filled. As a coach, I find my classes might be nailed down in terms of timings but everything around it is down to me to sort out.

While I loved the dynamism that came with working for a pioneering venture like Peloton, I didn't want to repeat my negative experience on the graduate scheme and risk becoming overwhelmed. This is where I leaned on and utilised the life coach that I was using at the time. Together, we devised strategies for making sure I was efficient and in control of both my professional and personal life. I learned to manage my own diary while building in flexibility so I could react to tasks without being swamped. It was a revelation, teaching me never to hold back when it comes to asking for help.

Whenever I have something on my mind, I talk to Leanne. She's great at putting things into perspective, and I hope I can do the same for her. We're so lucky to be in the same role as Peloton instructors. We have had totally different life experiences, yet we share very similar roles now. We make a great team, and it's one that's unique.

As a couple, only Leanne and I know how it feels when a Peloton class goes live around the world or just how important it is to find peace and quiet at the end of a demanding day. As the platform has grown, we've become familiar faces to the community. We both love that connectivity, but as in any area of public life, it can also bring an intense level of interest or scrutiny. It means that we have to think about anything we say or do as only we are accountable for it. I've come to see that as a good thing. If I aim to be kind and considerate in everything I do, then surely I can't have any regrets?

In terms of wellbeing, I also find it helps to ensure I always hold back time to myself. I set myself boundaries and value that privacy. That way, if my work attracts negative attention on social media, for example, I can switch off from it. There's a big difference between constructive criticism, which is a learning opportunity, and comments that are just intended to cause upset or humiliation. I've learned to ignore the latter, simply by unplugging on a regular basis and reminding myself of what's important. In my view, if you stay totally and authentically true to yourself and do everything with the right intentions, then you will have nothing to regret or hide. It's a liberating feeling to live out your authentic self, while gravitating towards the people who bring you good energy and moving away from those who don't.

People sometimes ask me if I look back on my finance career as a wasted opportunity. As far as I'm concerned, it was a vital stepping stone. I may no longer be sitting behind a desk for 10 to 14 hours a day, but my experience in dealing with business issues is still useful to me. As Peloton has grown in reach and scope, I've found myself increasingly involved in meetings and teams working on how to bring Peloton to the next level. Innovation and growth are things that drive me, and I am constantly thinking about how we can take things up a gear. Whether it's designing a new class model or securing a deal with a new artist for a memorable collaboration, I've discovered that my early years in finance haven't gone to waste. Whenever we start talking about numbers, strategies and corporate issues, I'm on it!

Above all, I have found that adaptation is key to making the most of life. None of us are born to be great at anything. We have to learn and practise skills, and then take them to another level if we want to excel. It's here that I truly believe in the power of continued learning. More and more of us are going to the gym and looking after our bodies these days, but are we working out our minds?

At the time of writing, I'm in the process of building my knowledge in nutrition and functional medicine, and have taken numerous additional fitness qualifications over the years to level up my coaching. Don't wait for your work to send you on a course. In this world of hybrid and fluid career paths, a drive and openness to learn new things is key to success in the future.

Even if we master a subject or skill, only to move on to other interests, that knowledge or experience is often transferable. It's a journey, but we all have to start somewhere and that point can make or break us. Why? Because starting out in any pursuit or passion can be intimidating. It's easy to feel like we have no right to be there, and then walk away before we've even begun. In work or play, when we take on a new challenge it will always shine a light on our experience (or lack of it). It's here we need the self-belief to remind ourselves that we can master whatever situation we're in, but it takes time, support and dedication.

From hosting club nights and running an investment society to coaching my first indoor cycling class, I had no experience to call upon in any of these fields when I began. Instead, I have learned that passion counts for everything as we find our feet, along with a willingness to learn – not just from knowledge but setbacks and mistakes. That way, over time we come into our own. Sometimes I look back at my short career in finance and wonder if I could have made it a long-term success. I was out of my depth to begin with and, though it threatened to drag me down, I strived to stay afloat. Had I stuck it out, I dare say I might have learned to swim. I'm glad I won't find out, however, because from the moment I entered those waters I knew they wouldn't make me happy.

Learning to become a fitness coach hasn't been easy. I felt like an imposter the first time I hosted a class and had to place my faith in Peloton when they saw potential in me that I hadn't necessarily registered myself. As an instructor, I had moments of self-doubt, as well as times when I knew that I could do better, but one thing differed from finance on that learning curve and it came down to the fact that I loved what I was doing. This is what drove me from the moment I started coaching. In any pursuit we set out to master, it underpins the mindset and energy required for success. A healthy dose of honesty and self-awareness is also part of the process, because this is how we learn to improve. I knew I had a long way to go on my journey in order to be my best self as a trainer. I'm just grateful to Peloton for inviting me to join them for the ride, along with Leanne, my family and friends for supporting me all the way.

After two years as a Peloton instructor, feeling at home on the platform and with the community, I decided it was time to own my cancer story. Until then, I had kept it only to family and friends. I was worried that somehow illness wouldn't sit right with the concept of health and fitness, but as time passed, I began to reflect on what had happened to me in a different light.

Without a doubt, coming through a serious illness has given me a renewed appreciation of life's joys and fragility. At the same time, it has left me somewhat wary of the sun. I take sensible precautions, as everyone should, and yet I'm still fearful about being out and about in strong sunlight. It's something I try to work on, but after what I went through it might be a permanent feature in my life, like the scar on my back. I realised that by withholding this chapter of my life from others, however, I wasn't presenting my true self in full. It was a version with a filter applied, and that didn't sit right with my values. I also recognised that I was in a position of some influence as a fitness instructor, and that brought with it a certain responsibility.

With this in mind, I decided that opening up about my experience might be helpful to others. When I told my team, I worried they might react like I had been withholding vital information. Instead, they showed me nothing but warmth and encouragement, and I realised that sharing my whole story just made me human. And since I've told my story publicly, there have been a number of people reaching out to say it has inspired them to get checked out, too. It feels good to know that sharing my story has given hope and support to others who are going through similar struggles.

*

GETTING TO GRIPS WITH GRATITUDE

There's a great deal to be said for being thankful in life. On a day-to-day basis, good manners are a quality that can create a positive first impression. It doesn't take much to acknowledge someone for holding a door, and yet, in that moment, such a small gesture can define who we are.

We all lead busy lives. If we've set out to challenge ourselves and push to be our best selves, then we could even see it as a sign that things are going well! At the same time, it's vital that we make space for ourselves. I'm not just talking about flopping in front of the TV at the end of a busy day, but being conscious of how fortunate we are to be leading the lives we choose to pursue. Through this lens, we can be grateful for the simplest things that we would otherwise take for granted – from a clear, sunny day to the discovery that there's just enough milk in the fridge to make a cup of tea. It might not sound like much, but it can be the starting point to fuel everything from our mindset and motivation to the quality of our character.

It would be wrong to think that placing gratitude at the forefront of our lives means we should be floating through each day with a smile pasted to our faces. It's simply about raising an awareness within ourselves that keeps our egos in check and reminds us of what's important in life. As a form of mindfulness, being thankful can only be a positive force that supports our mental health and strengthens relationships with everyone in our lives, from family and friends to colleagues, clients and anybody who interacts with us on an everyday basis. We become individuals who celebrate the good rather than dwell upon the negative.

We all know how to be grateful, but sometimes we can fall out of the habit of practising it. A simple aim is to identify one thing each day for which to be thankful. As long as it comes from the heart, what starts out as a conscious and even awkward thought process can swiftly become second nature.

Showing gratitude isn't limited to the here and now. By looking back at our journey and recognising just how far we've come, we can be thankful for everything from the opportunities we faced, to the people who helped us overcome challenges. In essence, we're acknowledging all the formative experiences and strong relationships that we have forged along the way. As an affirmation, it's a source of positivity that encourages us to stay grounded and humble, while raising awareness of all that is good with our lives. Ultimately, showing gratitude is our way of recognising the value of happiness, which is what life is all about.

Working in the fitness space, I strive to remind myself how fortunate I am to be in good health. My body is the tool I need in order to work. It's a physical job, and I express my gratitude by staying in shape. It's a simple affirmation that comes to mind every time I host a class – and forms the basis for the energy I hope to bring. You never know who needs you. Positive energy is contagious. Every time I jump on the bike, I could be helping someone dig themselves out from a really dark day. This is my motivation and should be all of ours in whatever we do. Be mindful with what you are allowing into your space. Choose a new frequency. Negativity vibrates at a different frequency. Elevate and create positivity and the negatives will be out of your range.

For me, the act of being thankful has almost become a ritual. It's a fleeting moment, but sometimes it can mean so much to me. We all have challenges in our lives, after all, and so if I'm carrying the weight of the world on my shoulders, it's a means of reminding myself that I can still be thankful for the opportunities that life has presented me with.

Showing gratitude helps us to put everything in perspective. It lifts the spirit, reminds us of our values and centres us once again so that we can face the day as a force for good.

GOING BACK TO OUR ROOTS

Success can be a double-edged sword. It's something we all strive towards in some shape or form. Everyone has a different concept of what success means, of course. Whether it's recognition for our efforts, financial stability, a position of power, authority and influence or the top spot on a podium, we know it takes time, commitment, teamwork and sacrifice. In becoming successful, however, it's all too easy to lose sight of the journey that delivered us there.

Often, that disconnection is down to the demands that success can bring. The hard work doesn't always stop when we achieve our goals. If anything, it can encourage us to establish new targets and keep pushing. This is fine on one level, but it can encourage some to take their success for granted. As a result, we can forget to recognise the people who helped us to get where we are, or adopt an attitude that success is an entitlement rather than the result of what is almost always a collective effort.

We've all come across individuals in life who consider success to be a measure of their value as human beings. From the difficult boss to the celebrity with unreasonable demands, these stereotype characters are often based on a kernel of truth. Naturally, none of us want to fall into this mindset, and no doubt those who have already done so would be horrified by how it can feed into their reputation. This is something that everyone needs to consider. Humility isn't something we can create artificially. It comes down to embodying our values at all times, being humble no matter what our position and simply treating others with the same respect we hope to receive from them. A sense of gratitude brings these elements together and can serve as the reality check that we all need in order to remain at the top of our game for all the right reasons. In every case, this begins by acknowledging every step of the journey we've taken from the moment we set out.

Today, coaching on a global fitness platform, I can sometimes find myself in front of an audience that numbers tens, even hundreds of thousands. It's an incredible figure, and I remind myself every day how fortunate I am. I'm also well aware that I didn't just arrive at this moment overnight. That kind of instant success is largely a fairy tale that in reality happens to very few people. If I look back at my journey to Peloton, it quite possibly began on the football pitch, where I had my dad – who I consider to be my mentor – to thank for pushing me to the top of my game.

When I first started coaching indoor cycling classes on a casual basis, I could sometimes expect no more than six people at my early morning sessions. Nevertheless, I was so grateful to each and every one of them. They were showing up on a weekday before the sun had risen! Even when I joined the Peloton platform as it launched in the UK, our audience was a fraction of what it is now. In fact, I have a very clear memory of Leanne jumping for joy on discovering 150 people on her leader board. She was thrilled, as was I, and that buzz validated our efforts. Not only that, but it also renewed our commitment to keep pushing for the highest standards throughout every workout we host.

These are two of many milestones on my journey that I regularly reflect upon. Regardless of the numbers, the sense of achievement was immense, as was my gratitude to those who had made it happen. It means that when I find myself coaching a session on the platform with users from all across the globe, I am just as thankful to everyone present as I was to those six who showed up early in my career. It really is a blessing for me to have this chance to guide people on their fitness journey, and I never want to lose sight of that fact.

Alongside this outlook on my journey, I want to stay conscious of my privilege. I come from a comfortable background, with a solid education and, while I have always aimed to make the most of these opportunities, I am aware that they aren't open to everyone. It's a great leveller to remind myself of this on a regular basis; it encourages me to do my best at all times in recognition that I am fortunate to follow this path in life.

RECOGNISING THE TEAM

When a Formula One racing driver steps up onto the podium at the end of a gruelling race, it's undeniably their moment of glory. They've fought hard for an advantage around countless laps of a track that can be measured in one-hundredths of a second and deserve to be celebrated for their efforts. At the same time, it would be easy to overlook the fact that the driver isn't solely responsible for the victory. Behind the scenes, a whole team of individuals with specialist skills, from the race engineers to the catering crew, have played a critical role. The driver is the first to recognise this, which is why in the post-race interview they always share the credit for the win and thank everyone involved for making their dream come true.

We might not be Formula One drivers, but whatever pursuit we have embraced in life is rarely a solo venture. From the moment we start our journey – and we could be talking about life here – we rely on other people at different stages and in different ways. It isn't just about those who lend a helping hand, but individuals who teach us skills, provide emotional support and encourage us to take on challenges when we're doubting ourselves. From family and friends, teachers, colleagues, fellow players and even those who inspire us who we've never met, we all have a team behind us.

It pays to acknowledge that our success is down to a team effort. No matter how indirect the input, there are people out there who helped us to get where we are. We might take on a venture that demands time away from the family. Yes, we're pushing at our limits, but let's not forget our partner back home who is holding the fort in our absence. Without them, we wouldn't be in a position to pursue that dream. By recognising this, and being thankful for the role that everyone played, we can only grow as individuals. It means we don't buy into an oversized sense of our own importance and instead stay humble and also connected with reality. Acknowledging our team doesn't take away from any success or achievement we might have made. If anything, by celebrating together it enhances the experience.

I only have to look back at my life in fitness to register the team effort that contributes to my role. I might be the face on the screen in a Peloton coaching session, but the reality is there are hundreds of people hard at work behind the scenes to make it happen. I am just a cog in an efficient machine. I perform the public-facing task, but in my view it's no more important than any other job in the Peloton ecosystem. What's more, I am keenly aware that, when Peloton first launched in the UK, I could count the team members on one hand. We all pulled together to make each workout happen, and that demanded flexibility from me as much as everyone else. We just got on and did whatever had to be done. We were driven by a shared commitment and passion for the vision of bringing a gym fitness session into the home and, as that became a reality, so the team grew to support it.

I feel so fortunate to have been part of this journey for so long. In seeing the platform develop, I have never lost sight of where we began and the people who made it happen. Being surrounded by a great team brings so many benefits. That shared sense of adventure can be hugely motivating. Knowing you can trust the people around you can also increase your appetite for risk. By pooling together our skills, knowledge and support, we can aim higher, dream bigger and achieve things that might not be possible alone. A team can be in the background or standing shoulder to shoulder with us for the winning photograph. Either way, being grateful for everything they have done can be the binding force that propels us forward as one.

KICKING COMPLACENCY INTO TOUCH

We know that gratitude can remind us of the road to our achievements, including the wins along the way as well as the team that made it happen. There is another benefit to being mindful of the undertaking we have made, and that comes down to its role as an antidote to complacency.

For most of us, success does not come easily. It demands hard work, time and commitment, and when we reach the summit that sense of elation can be matched by exhaustion. As a measure of the effort we've made, it's completely understandable. Issues only arise if we fail to rest in order to help recover and grow from the experience, but instead become comfortable on that pinnacle. As a result, we lose focus on future challenges, and put in the minimum effort to maintain our position. In truth, we become lazy, and that has a cascading effect on the team that worked alongside us in our ascent to the top.

By remaining aware of our journey and being thankful for the experience and the opportunities we've grasped, it's very hard for us to be complacent. We can't take anything for granted when we know what's behind our success, and that keeps us from sitting back. It's about staying wise to the effort and making sure that we relax at the right moment and for the right reasons. Everyone deserves time out. What matters is that we use it to enjoy life and recharge, rather than stay in the driving seat and slowly let our foot off the gas.

Checking in with our roots plays such an important role in our continued progress. It reminds us that we set out with a passion and keeps it burning brightly. It can also help us to stay at the top of our game. Whenever I'm invited to speak in public, at an event or as a guest on a podcast, I remind myself just how much it meant to me when I first stood in front of the school assembly to address the hall. I was so nervous, which was entirely natural, and with experience I learned to control those feelings and even use them as a force to keep me on my toes. Today, whenever I'm lucky enough to be addressing an audience,

I remind myself of just how far out of my comfort zone I used to feel in this environment. I might be more comfortable with it now, but that memory is enough to be sure that I make the same effort as I did on that first attempt. Without that reminder, which is enough to quicken my heartbeat, I would draw breath to speak and sound like I was half asleep. Looking at gratitude in this light, as a reminder that experience can lead to complacency, it becomes another tool in our kit that we can use to stay sharp.

Age is a factor that we must all consider as our journey continues. As the years mount up behind us, it's tempting to feel like that's where our best work lies. We see younger people come into play, who bring an energy that can be hard to match. Often, this leads to veterans in the field becoming complacent as they no longer feel like they can compete. This is a shame, because experience brings a certain quality that's often not available to us when we first start out, and that's wisdom.

My dad is a case in point. He's a rare breed in finance, having spent his entire career on the trading floor. As I saw for myself as a boy, with high hopes of following in his footsteps, it's a fast-paced, high-risk environment, and not one where I personally would have thrived. In a senior position now, my dad can count on colleagues who are my age. They're smart and quick to act on trades, whereas my dad brings a different game to the table. He's been there for so long that he's seen it all before. Nothing is unprecedented for him, which makes him unique in the team. He knows the DNA of the business because he represents it! As a result, the combination of energy and experience that comes from different generations is hard to beat, and that keeps my old man motivated long into his career.

GIVING BACK

Now we come to an aspect of grateful living that can prove to be infinitely rewarding. Having worked so hard to make the most of our lives, from pursuing dreams and creating opportunities to building resilience to overcome obstacles, we can look back on our journey and appreciate the transformation. We started out with high hopes and acquired wisdom and experience in the process. Whatever our definition of success, we find ourselves in a position that can seem far out of reach for those who hope to follow in our footsteps.

Many in this situation donate to charity, and let's be in no doubt that this can be a vital means of providing help and support to sectors of our society that need it most. At the same time, it's worth broadening our definition of what giving back means, because we can also deliver meaningful help and support in other ways.

As a schoolboy footballer, I was sometimes asked to help coach younger players and I loved it. It felt like a real privilege – and it was such a buzz to see kids pick up the skills I shared with them. The experience really made a mark on me. As a fitness coach with a public profile, I'm often contacted by people just starting out in the same field who are seeking advice on how to establish their careers. It's flattering to be asked, and I want to help if I can. While I can't provide shortcuts to success, I can answer questions that build confidence or offer insight into what can seem like a daunting challenge. I also remember how it felt to be in their situation and, indeed, when I first started to seriously consider coaching as my calling I asked as many questions as I could. I was so grateful to those who provided me with answers, and always vowed that if I ever made it then I would do the same.

Giving, like gratitude, can be a great source of personal enrichment. It allows us to acknowledge the journey we've undertaken and be thankful for a life well lived.

GRATITUDE FOR LIFE

We don't need to wait until we've found success before looking back in gratitude. It's a quality we should express throughout our journey, because, from the moment we make that first step, we have reason to be thankful. It's a privilege to create a vision of where we want to be and then align ourselves to pursuing it. We know that journey won't always be easy, and in aiming high we should expect difficulties and setbacks that truly test our character.

Life isn't always that simple. Sometimes, events can threaten to derail our plans, but by staying grounded and counting on our team at challenging times, we can only get through stronger for the experience. For that alone, we should be grateful, as much as for the opportunity to take control of our lives and raise the bar as high as we dare to dream.

RAISE THE BAR: MILESTONES

- Being thankful in life allows us to stay grounded, strengthens meaningful relationships, supports our mental health and encourages us to commit to being fit and active.
- If we're grateful for the success we create and mindful of the hard work it demanded and the opportunities we embraced, we'll never lose touch with our roots.
- Being aware of just how far we've come is an effective antidote to complacency. If life itself is a journey, let's make it fulfilling, every step of the way.

CREATING BALANCE AND MOTIVATION: A VISUAL EXERCISE

I intentionally wrote *Raise the Bar* without including lots of diagrams, graphs or infograms. However, to please my logical economics-graduate mind, I wanted to offer you a visual that serves as a reminder of the crucial aspects of your life requiring daily attention. These segments symbolise the elements that significantly influence your mental and physical wellbeing.

Given that we all have limited time and energy each day, week and month to dedicate to these areas, it's essential to occasionally assess and take stock of where we are spending time and energy. This self-reflection allows you to hold yourself accountable, readjust as necessary and achieve a harmonious balance that will help propel you towards success.

In the image overleaf, each segment corresponds to a specific area of your life that ideally warrants daily nurturing. The illustrated image shows all these elements evenly distributed. But let's be honest, these things are never all going to hold equal weight in your life at any one time. It will evolve across our lives but it's important to have awareness of where you're at now and of where you want to get to. Use a sheet of paper to create your own wheel, and personalise the size of each element for your current situation and your unique circumstances. Then use a second sheet of paper to create your ideal, redistributed balance, to remind yourself of where you want to get to. Try to link this back to your five-minute action or commitment (see page 47) to ensure you're taking steps towards it every day.

I recommend placing this image of your ideal wheel in a prominent place that you frequently refer to, enabling you to update it whenever your life undergoes shifts and changes. Each item within the image serves as either an inspiration or a prompt, encouraging you to take actions that may foster growth and wellbeing in those particular areas.

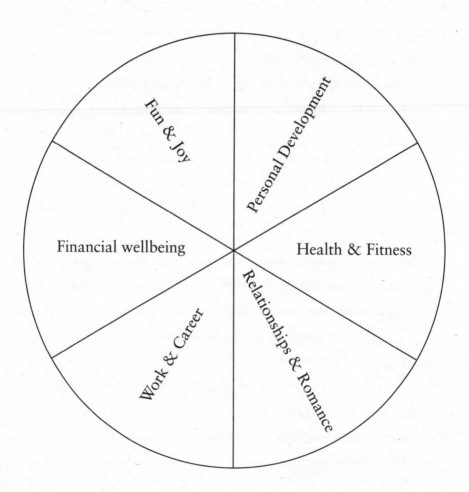

EPILOGUE

RIDE FOR LIFE

Life is a continuous journey of self-assessment
and self-evaluation, allowing us to alter our use of our time
and energy to prioritise what is important in life.

When I was asked to write this book, I felt daunted. Not least because my dyslexia makes reading and writing a challenge, and so, over the years, I've had to find workarounds and face that fear head on.

By sharing my beliefs, the systems I have put in place and the ways in which I have moved towards the life I want for myself, I was worried that it might seem like I was holding myself up as some kind of guru, one who has everything sorted and figured out.

I am not.

I have not.

Let's be honest, no one really has.

I was also concerned that it might seem to those facing daily battles in their lives that my choices and outlooks were trivial or blindly optimistic. Though I do strive for good choices, and optimism – like everyone, I hope – I can fall short in the course of 'real life'.

Please know that I by no means feel like I have it all figured out, but I *am* passionate about these principles and am evangelical about the ways in which tapping into my core values and bringing my mind and body into a good place by my own standards have helped me. That's day-to-day, as I move through life, and also in the face of my own personal challenges which have called everything into question.

My aim in writing *Raise the Bar* is to put the sum total of my experience and knowledge into actionable advice and strategies, and an outlook that can help us to live our best lives. I believe in every word I have shared, but of course it's only right to recognise that sometimes reality can determine how that plays out. We are humans after all, with individual needs, responsibilities, interests and pressures. I might endeavour to embody my values and beliefs, but then days happen when things don't go to plan. I feel it's important to recognise that and not be too hard on ourselves if we fall short. Life is a continuous journey of self-assessment and self-evaluation, allowing us to alter our use of our time and energy to prioritise what is important in life.

No growth is linear and the best-laid plans and dreams can get derailed at any time. The true test is how we deal with those setbacks. Writing this book has given me space to see that, without the tools and foundations that I've shared here, I might not have been able to face the challenges that have been thrown at me and my family over the past few years.

As I'm sure many people can relate to, during the global pandemic

I experienced enormous amounts of health anxiety. I felt constant stress about my health and my loved ones catching Covid-19 and the unknowns around how long this world crisis might go on for. This stress led to me having crippling anxiety daily that impacted on me physically and mentally. Instead of acknowledging this and taking steps to help myself, this often led to me drinking too much alcohol, eating fast food and not looking after myself away from the camera.

My job and main focus at the time was to help and inspire others to stay fit and healthy, but ironically during this period I wasn't practising what I preached, and wasn't finding the motivation and time to do for myself what I was encouraging others to do. I was choosing to put all my energy into what felt safe to me, filming content in our home studio and staying home with Leanne, away from the potential of catching Covid-19. I was slowly but surely distancing myself from the outside world and, as the world started to open up, I found myself not wanting to get back out there.

If I'm honest, I haven't been the same since. I am still struggling to rebuild a lot of the friendships and relationships I had prior to the pandemic. I still have periods of anxiety and stress like never before. This period of my life was a huge time of growth for me and pushed me to tackle my mental health challenges head on, but there are still many knock-on effects that I am processing.

The reason why this concluding chapter is so incredibly important to me is that, while writing this book, life changed a lot for me. A series of events took place that altered my perspective on so many things, made me question my own life choices and taught me some valuable lessons. Some of the toughest moments in our lives have the opportunity to either break us or build us up into the strongest and most resilient people we can be.

*

As the UK began a phased approach to exiting lockdown in July 2021, the opportunity to travel again became a possible reality. After spending so much time with Leanne during the lockdown, we were closer than ever and I knew by this stage that I wanted to ask her to marry me. I had known this for a while in fact, but Covid-19 had got in the way of that thinking. Deep down, I'm a bit of a hopeless romantic and I wanted to make sure the proposal was one to remember and not just me asking Leanne to marry me in our home.

The first country to open its borders was Spain and, with Ibiza being Leanne's favourite holiday destination, it seemed a no-brainer that we would try to book a trip away. And so, the grand proposal plan started to develop. Fortunately, everything ran smoothly, from me asking her dad, to getting the ring made, to flights and hotels not being cancelled at the last moment, to Covid tests being negative, and so I was able to ask Leanne to marry me on the second day of our trip.

I went all out and rented the amphitheatre at our hotel, which was located in a picturesque and private spot in the middle of mountains, with the most incredible view of the ocean. I had asked the hotel to lay out white petals on the walkway down and had her favourite bottle of champagne on ice at the table that had been set up so we could have a drink together and toast our future – after she hopefully said 'yes'. Thankfully, it all went to plan and asking my best friend to marry me was one of the best moments of my life so far.

After arriving home, Leanne and I were on top of the world and decided to throw a big engagement party to celebrate with our friends and family. Things were beginning to look up and I was starting to reconnect with my friends and family again. I had clocked back into the mindset of taking care of my mind and body and was feeling more comfortable getting out in public again. This was the well-needed shove for me to build up the confidence to get back out into the world.

The next year was all about navigating a new normal of being engaged and figuring out what was next for the both of us. We started talking about starting a family together and set our sights on buying our first home. After months of looking, we came across the perfect place for us. We were the first to view it and put in an offer right away. After a couple of weeks of back and forth with the estate agent and Leanne sending the owners a letter and a gift explaining why we would be the perfect fit to take care of the home that they had built, our offer was accepted and the process of buying our house began. For anyone who has gone through this process before, it's a mammoth task and doing this alongside a busy schedule at Peloton was the catalyst for lots of additional anxiety. But regardless, we were buying our first home together and we were so incredibly excited.

Summer 2022 was the summer of weddings.

All the weddings that were supposed to happen during the lockdown years were now taking place and lots of Leanne's and my friends were getting married. The wedding that everyone was looking forward to that summer was that of Danielle, Leanne's best friend since she'd started her professional dance career back in the early 2000s, to her partner, Tom, an incredible singer-songwriter. Pretty much all our friends were invited. Our friends love any excuse to have a party and always dress to impress, so there was no doubt this was going to be an event to remember.

It was a boiling hot day, none of us will forget the heat that day, and, as I was on my way to the venue with some of my friends, I received a message from Leanne that changed our lives for ever. She was a bridesmaid and was with Danielle getting ready for her big day, when the day took a turn that still doesn't feel real. Danielle suddenly became unwell, collapsed and devastatingly passed away less than 24 hours later. From that day onwards, our lives have never been the same. They never will again.

This horrendously shocking and devastatingly sad event ripped through our friendship group and hit Leanne like a tonne of bricks. She had lost her best friend on her wedding day. Her grief has been heartbreaking to see. Nothing can prepare you for dealing with something as traumatic as this. Nothing prepares you for something so sad.

I was doing my best to support Leanne but was still trying to keep some normality and teach classes at Peloton. Leanne was understandably distraught and took some time away from work, but I threw myself into it. A coping mechanism most likely.

In the weeks prior to the wedding, Leanne and I had exchanged on our dream home. We were in the process of decorating it and had been getting it ready to move all our stuff in when Danielle and Tom's wedding day came. We never got the opportunity to celebrate the move in with each other, as the main focus during that time was supporting each other in the lead up to the funeral.

*

Two days before that dreaded day, Leanne and I were in bed together, when she bolted and ran into the bathroom. She screamed at me:

'I've got a lump in my boob. Ben, I've got a lump in my boob! F**K F**K F**K.'

In absolute shock and disbelief, I tried to stay calm and got up, asking her if I could feel it. Despite having limited medical knowledge, I could feel the small lump, but not well, so I tried to calm Leanne down by saying it was probably nothing. She didn't calm down.

'Let's get you booked in to see the doctor as soon as possible and you can get it checked,' I said as reassuringly as I could.

We managed to book her an appointment with a private GP and, a couple of hours later, she went. She messaged me as soon as she got out of the clinic to say they weren't that worried and thought it was a hormonal cyst. They told her that if it was still there in a couple of weeks to come back to get a referral for further checks. Leanne was by no means convinced, but at least they hadn't confirmed the worst and her focus could be on the funeral without additional anxiety about her own health.

A couple of weeks passed and the lump still hadn't gone away. Having had cancer myself in my early twenties, I knew that the smartest thing to do at this stage was for Leanne to go and get a scan done to rule out the worst. I encouraged her to book an appointment as soon as possible and they booked her into a breast cancer clinic to have it looked at. Because it was so last-minute, I couldn't get out of work and Leanne had to go on her own. At this point, we still thought it was a hormonal cyst and she was just going to the doctor to rule out anything worse.

Later, when I was in the studio at work, as I finished filming, I collected my phone and saw a message pop up from Leanne:

Ben, you need to get here now.

Panicked and worried, I grabbed my stuff and rushed to the hospital. As I arrived, Leanne texted me where to come, directing me to the room where she sat alongside a doctor and two nurses. She was incredibly upset and the doctor explained to me that they had done the scans and that they thought they had found cancerous cells in one of her breasts. Once more, our whole world was turned upside down in just a moment.

Neither of us could believe what we were hearing. Shocked, we just looked at each other in despair. I felt awful that I had let Leanne go to the hospital alone. We were then taken into a separate room and had the opportunity to speak to a cancer nurse who explained the next steps – that they would send away the biopsy sample they had taken for testing and would see us again in a week's time for a follow-up. The nurse gave us leaflets to explain the different types of breast cancer and the potential treatment options. If I'm honest, I cannot remember a lot of what she said. We both walked out of the hospital numb, dreading the 'follow-up'.

I've sat in a room myself and been diagnosed with cancer, so to an extent I could recognise the fear in Leanne. I was offered the job at Peloton not long after recovering from my surgery, and because I didn't really take the necessary time to process the emotions and feelings that I felt during that period of my own life, I felt like I was reliving it, but this time through the woman I had asked to marry me, a woman already dealing with so much.

Another week went by and after the follow-up with the consultant, Leanne was diagnosed with Grade 3 triple positive breast cancer. The likelihood of having to go through chemotherapy, surgery and radiotherapy was very high and that is where we, as a family, had to go into fight or flight mode and tackle this head on.

Cancer is as much a mental challenge as it is a physical one. This is what one of Leanne's cancer nurses told us just after she was diagnosed. It consumes you and pushes you to question the strength of your own mind and body. I needed to and was going to do everything within my power to help her fight this, while maintaining a positive mindset throughout. Leanne was my top priority and we were going to beat this together.

What attracted me to Leanne when I first met her was her carefree and sparkly attitude to life. She is the epitome of someone who lives life to the fullest. She has always worked incredibly hard, having toured around the word as a professional dancer for many years prior to Peloton, and she has this amazing ability to light up any room she walks into. If anyone was going to tackle this head on, it was her – and with me and the rest of her family by her side, we were a pretty solid team. We threw ourselves into learning everything about the treatment process and started working out how we could support her to the best of our ability.

It was confirmed Leanne would need chemotherapy, surgery, radiotherapy, and the likely impact on her fertility meant that before she started her treatment, we were advised to go through the IVF process to try and freeze some embryos. We were incredibly lucky to be successful, but it was another curveball that we weren't prepared for. Left with little to no option, we faced it head on together.

*

As I write this, Leanne has been going through treatment. I am incredibly proud of her for how she has handled herself throughout. She has maintained focus in times during which most would have crumbled. She has stayed positive in times when most would have fallen into despair. And she has tackled every step of the process with a determination that has inspired me to be a better person myself.

She continued to show up to teach her classes week by week at Peloton. Every Wednesday during her chemotherapy treatment, she would start her day by heading to the studio for her early-morning classes and then go straight to the hospital for treatment, showing up for others, even at times when that was all the energy she could manage in a day. An absolute inspiration to all of us, Leanne has made everyone who knows her stronger as people. If she can do what she is doing while she is going through what she is facing, then we can do anything. I can.

It's fair to say the last year has been cruel to us both. Losing Danielle so suddenly and tragically, and then straight afterwards Leanne receiving the diagnosis of breast cancer, has resulted in a rollercoaster of emotions. I've been terrified, but have tried to maintain as much normality away from the hospital appointments to stay hopeful and do my best to help us both fulfil our day-to-day roles – to continue being Peloton instructors, good partners, good friends, a good son/daughter, brother/sister, auntie/uncle.

Leanne has taken every step of this journey in her stride, with so much grace and with her head held high. Through countless hospital appointments for IVF treatments, chemotherapy, surgery, weeks of radiotherapy, check-ups, scans and injections – every second of the way – I have been proud to stand by her side and she has demonstrated tenfold to me why I am so incredibly lucky that she said yes to marrying me.

We have certainly said 'F*** You' to cancer countless times with the actions we have taken over the last 12 months and, while we're not out of the woods, I am incredibly happy, euphoric, that, as I write this book's last chapter, Leanne has finished the main bulk of her treatment and has been given the positive news that she no longer has cancer in her body. While she is still undergoing preventative treatment, which she will continue on with for many years to come, she has done it! She has beaten cancer. She absolutely smashed it!

It's important to note that the road to recovery isn't over and it will be a long and hard process for Leanne to build her mind and body back up, but in times like this you have to celebrate the wins, regardless of their size.

So here's to, as Leanne would say, 'sparkly days ahead' and 'living our healthiest and happiest lives', using countless lessons that the last year has taught us, but particularly me.

I have been forced to grow and learn fast in the past few years. The challenges that have been thrown my way have tested me both physically and mentally. The resilience that I have managed to build and life lessons that I have learned along the way combine as a superpower I hold close to my heart. I know, with certainty, that if I've made it through some of the most challenging moments I have had to navigate in the last few years, I can tackle anything that is thrown my way. I have no doubts about that.

I think it's imperative to say that, without some of the tools I have broken down in this book, there is no way I would have been able to handle the pressures and things thrown at me, especially recently. And this is the very reason why I am so passionate about sharing the importance of us all working on building a mentally and physically strong mind and body to prepare us for whatever life throws our way.

Writing this book has allowed me to figure a lot of this stuff out and get down on paper a structure to help me continue to build a healthy and happy life for myself – and my loved ones – going forward. I'm now on a mission to share these tools to help you and millions like you do the same.

Regardless of where you feel you are in your life, you are not alone. We are all still learning as we go. Some people will face challenges that will force them to grow and develop; others choose to put themselves in challenging situations to help them develop and grow. The most important lessons I have learned have all come from some of the toughest moments I have faced. Those periods of challenge have changed me as a person and given me a new perspective on life and where my priorities lie.

We will never have it all figured out though. That is what makes the quest of life so amazing. Many of the most important lessons can't be learned in a self-help book or textbooks; the brutal truth is we need to get out there and experience the good, the bad and the ugly first-hand.

We need to navigate through uncertainty to come out the other side more resilient and stronger than ever. Hopefully, the tools I have gifted you in this book will aid you on that journey. It's amazing to think that some of our best days in life haven't happened yet. Here's to RAISING THE BAR for ourselves, living out the happiest and healthiest lives and making memories alongside our loved ones.

ACKNOWLEDGEMENTS

Writing a book is harder than I ever thought and more rewarding than I could have ever imagined. None of this would have been possible without my sparkly fiancée Leanne. We have been through so many highs and lows together across the last few years and I wouldn't be half the man I am today without your friendship, love and support. Your resilience and mental strength through health issues, career challenges, house moves, loss, grief and much more have been nothing but inspiring and I am lucky to have such a strong woman standing in my corner. Your *very* honest feedback on every aspect of my life has shaped me into a better man and I can't wait to continue sharing the rest of my life with you.

I'm eternally grateful to my mum, who spent countless hours with me as a child asking the most random questions and teaching me the importance of being open with my emotions. I am hugely thankful to my dad, who taught me the importance of working hard, competitive spirit and building a future for yourself and your family.

To my three sisters, Jenny, Emma and Sophie, thank you for putting up with me as the only boy in a four-child household (often labelling me as the favourite child). You allowed me to learn and navigate through the good and challenging times of family life.

To my late grandad, Bert, and nan, Val, who opened up my eyes to the importance of family, community and helping others, plus encouraged me to explore the world and celebrated every success of mine, however big or small. I hope I have made you proud Grandad. I miss you ever so much.

To my publisher Briony Gowlett and the Radar team, thank you for seeing the potential in this book and helping me bring it to life. Briony, you are an absolute rock star. You have pushed me to grow more, and it's been the most incredible experience writing this book alongside you.

To my co-author Matt Whyman, you are an absolute legend my friend. Straight from the off, we clicked and you understood where we wanted to take this book. You are amazing at what you do, and I am forever grateful for the time, hard work and guidance you gave to get this book to where it is today.

To the Peloton and Ben's Army community, you have demonstrated time and time again how powerful the 'Together We Go Far' mentality can be. You have shown up and showed support through the good, the bad and the ugly since I joined Peloton in 2018, and for that I am incredibly grateful. This is just the beginning of this wonderful journey together. We didn't come this far to only get this far, right? Thank you, and I believe the best is still yet to come!

Finally, to all my friends, colleagues, teachers, study partners, clients, teammates, sports coaches, lecturers and bosses I've met and worked with along the way. I am grateful for every experience, relationship, hard conversation, win, loss, laugh and tear we got to share together. Life has an incredible way of bringing the right people into your life at the right times (if you're open to it) and you have all had a part to play in mine, so thank you.

ABOUT THE AUTHOR

Ben Alldis is a London-based fitness and health expert, currently working at Peloton as a cycle and strength instructor. He joined the Peloton team, as the first UK-based male instructor, in 2018. Combining this with his previous experience working in finance and as a DJ, Ben sits at the intersection of fitness, business, tech, music, sports and entertainment. As a world-class Peloton instructor, a NASM-certified personal trainer and qualified nutrition coach, Ben is a unique hybrid of high-performance athlete and motivational coach. *Raise the Bar* is his first book.